TELEMEDICINE AND TELEHEALTH 2.0
A PRACTICAL GUIDE FOR MEDICAL PROVIDERS
AND PATIENTS

Victor Lyuboslavsky

ISBN: 1515135705
ISBN-13: 978-1515135708

Table of Contents

Acknowledgements

Many people helped and contributed a significant amount of time to the creation of this book. My wife, Yulia Lyuboslavsky, RN-BSN, MSN, ACNS-BC, provided much-needed emotional support and reviewed multiple drafts. My parents, Alexander Panov, MD, PhD, and Polina Lyuboslavsky, provided advice. My friend and business partner Cliff Sze, PhD, gave guidance based on his writing experience. My **md Portal** co-founders Paul Robichaux and Venessa Peña-Robichaux, MD shared insights into dermatology and the healthcare industry. Other people who helped include Health Wildcatters alumni, staff, and mentors; Capital Factory partners and mentors; md Portal customers; and friends.

Preface

Healthcare is the next frontier where we'll see considerable change and improvements in the next several decades. At its core we have a paradox – we want to provide the best possible care to everyone at the lowest possible price, all while the standard for best possible care continues to climb every year. Additional legal administration is not the answer. As Thomas Sowell, a well-known economist, says: "It is amazing that people who think we cannot afford to pay for doctors, hospitals, and medication somehow think that we can afford to pay for doctors, hospitals, medication and a government bureaucracy to administer it." To solve the dual challenges of higher quality care and more affordable care, we will need many innovations from the minds of the best and brightest medical professionals and engineers. Healthcare is truly the best industry to make a difference.

I co-founded **md Portal** http://mdPortal.com along with my co-founders Paul Robichaux and Venessa Peña-Robichaux, MD. We want to advance the delivery of healthcare for both patients and doctors. We're accomplishing this through telemedicine technologies. Fundamentally, md Portal tackles the issue of making high quality healthcare affordable for everyone. We sell our products to physician practices, and we provide the necessary tools to increase overall practice efficiency while maintaining the standard of quality care.

Writing this book is a continuation of our vision to advance the delivery of healthcare. We believe we're on the cusp of a massive transition to telemedicine, and we want all providers and patients to have this knowledge in their hands. Much of the content of the book is based on my conversation with my co-founders and other medical professionals. Throughout the book, I use the term "we" because the ideas and concepts in this book are not mine alone, but the result of accumulated wisdom from many people in the telemedicine and healthcare space.

All too often in recent history telemedicine deployments have failed because the project leaders did not know what to expect and what was involved. Telemedicine has been a buzzword and marketed as a magic pill to help cure all the issues in the healthcare system. And, although successes in telemedicine are mounting, we want all the stakeholders, medical providers, medical staff, and patients, to go into their telemedicine transition knowing exactly what to expect. We provide a realistic look at what's going on in telemedicine, both the considerable benefits telemedicine brings as well as the potential challenges to overcome. We do not sugar coat our experiences. All the examples are real, although some of the details have been changed for privacy. We want you, the reader, to know what to expect when using telemedicine and to make a good decision whether telemedicine is right for you.

As the Chief Technology Officer at md Portal, I'm responsible for scaling our telemedicine technologies across clinic locations, healthcare systems, and different specialties. I'm an engineer by trade, so parts of this book may have a slight technical leaning. Nevertheless, the goal has always been to make this material accessible for readers of any background. We are passionate about technology and human progress, and we're always excited to hear what's new in the world. A couple times a month, we like to take a step back, look at the world as a whole, and take an hour or two to brainstorm technological solutions and process improvements to the biggest issues of the day. On a personal note, the act of writing this book has helped me crystallize my thoughts and gain a much deeper appreciation of all the facets and possibilities that telemedicine brings to the table.

Introduction

Telemedicine is the ability to provide medical advice and treatment remotely. The prefix *tele* comes from ancient Greek and means: at a distance, far off, far away, or far from. In the past half-century, the prefix *tele* has also begun to be used for things related to television, such as telecast, for example. Hence, some people, upon hearing the term telemedicine, automatically assume that it refers to providing medical advice over television. In fact, telemedicine can be provided over any communication medium, and not just video.

As part of our day-to-day operations at md Portal, we speak to medical providers, healthcare professionals, and patients. One message we frequently hear is that **Telemedicine is the future**. Yes, we wholeheartedly agree with that assessment. Yet we want to take this sentiment a step further and ask: Why isn't Telemedicine "the present"? Why aren't you, as a medical provider, using the newer, more practical and efficient channels of telemedicine every day to provide medical care to your patients? And why aren't you, as a patient, asking your medical provider when they will have a telemedicine option for your regular follow-up? Why are so many people complaining about affordable access to care when we already know how to solve many of these issues?

After all, telemedicine technologies, the know-how, and the products are already here today. If we can connect most people on the globe via telephone, then surely we can connect patients with their physicians more efficiently. And yet that's not what we see. Even office managers and physicians who proclaim that telemedicine is the future are hesitant to start using telemedicine today. They need time to think, time to check whether their peers are using it, time to ask their patients about it, and time to figure out how to fit it into their existing processes. Numerous telemedicine companies have started up in the last two decades, and many have failed largely due to the difficulty of changing the existing physician-patient status quo, and due to the lack of buy-in from the medical community.

Now, let's not throw too much cold water on the fire. We're not here to talk about what can't be done, but about *what can be done* and *what is being done*. After all, you may have picked up this book to read about the wonders and magic of Telemedicine. And yes, the wonders are real. Technology is in place; telemedicine is relatively straightforward to set up; many health insurance companies are on board; and plenty of studies show that telemedicine provides quality healthcare. Part of the hesitancy of some medical providers is due to the uncertainty of all that telemedicine entails. Our perception is that many medical providers truly want to have the choice of telemedicine available for their patients, even though they're not quite sure whether or when they will use it. With numerous telemedicine deployments under our belt, we are here to help with the process, give a realistic outlook regarding what to expect and what to watch out for, and provide recommendations regarding making a smooth transition and taking maximum advantage of telemedicine.

A friend of ours, let's call him Raj, studied engineering at a major university during the 1980's. He was looking for roommates and decided to live with a couple of medical students. Since he spent a lot of time with them, they were frequently talking about the process of treating patients. Since Raj was a young and energetic fellow at the time, he decided to flex his engineering brain and apply some technology to the problems in healthcare.

He decided to focus on questionnaires. When patients come to see their medical provider with an issue, their provider asks them a series of questions to determine the patient's diagnosis. Most of the time, physicians see similar types of medical issues day in and day out. And, with experience, physicians develop their own routine series of questions to efficiently get to the bottom of the most common issues. So, Raj thought, why can't this process be automated with computers? After all, automating the patient interview could go a lot faster for both medical providers and their patients. Medical providers, especially, would save a lot of time by not having to repeat the same questions over and over to different patients, and then listening to the same types of responses. As one medical provider told us, "most of the time I know what the patient is going to say."

So, Raj decided to create a computer program to conduct the patient interview for primary care. He spoke to physicians, nurses, and medical staff. He built multiple paper prototypes of the questionnaire. The key feature of the program was the ability to ask the patient a different question based on their previous response. He wrote the program for a PDP-11 minicomputer made by the now defunct Digital Equipment Corporation (DEC). Back in the day, before the personal computer and Apple, DEC made many of the computers used by large corporations.

Raj's program worked. Raj's friends and potential patients used the program, went through the interview steps, and were amazed that the program spit out an accurate list of potential diagnoses. Aimed with the print out of all the answers, a medical provider could use that information to accurately diagnose the patient's issue most of the time.

This technology was way ahead of its time. Remember, it was the 1980's – medical clinics did not use computers and many patients have never even seen a computer. But, at the core of it, this was the asynchronous telemedicine – technology that is only now being used on a regular basis in healthcare. A patient, using a computer, fills out a questionnaire asking them about their condition. The paper print out is sent to a remote doctor (in a different room, building, or city), and the physician responds back with a medical diagnosis and prescriptions.

The technologies surrounding telemedicine are solid. Smart engineers have been thinking about assisting the healthcare industry with technology for a very long time. Many of today's engineers even consider telemedicine to be extremely simple -- put up some online forms and hook up a video camera or take pictures. And yes, the basics are simple. The challenge is streamlining the telemedicine deployment so that it provides overwhelming value.

Several process changes and integration technologies are involved in properly streamlining a telemedicine deployment. Humans, in general, are resistant to change. In addition, making changes when it comes to patient safety and the treatment of medical conditions is not to be taken lightly. After all, that's why pharmaceutical companies and medical device manufacturers often spend decades and huge sums of money on clinical trials, approval processes and marketing. In order to be embraced, telemedicine must show a definitive advantage for medical providers, patients, and investors. Two major drivers of change for both medical providers and patients are better medical care and financial benefits. As patients, we all want quality care and we want it to be cheap. Medical providers, on the other hand, want to help as many people as they can, given the current constraints of their availability, and keeping overhead costs as low as possible.

Rapid Adoption of Telemedicine

Fortunately, telemedicine is being adopted rapidly, with double-digit growth in the US telemedicine market expected through 2020. [1] The key drivers of telemedicine growth are:

- High-deductible insurance plans
- Risk-based reimbursement contracts and reimbursement cuts
- Increasing reimbursement and licensing expansion for telemedicine
- Switch to paperless medical records
- High overhead costs for medical providers

With the acceptance of health savings accounts (HSAs) and Affordable Care Act (ACA), also known as Obamacare, more and more patients are using high-deductible insurance plans. These plans typically have much lower premiums than traditional health insurance plans. The low premiums are attractive for patients, especially for younger ones, even though they come with higher co-pays and deductibles. What this means is that these types of patients are price sensitive to the costs of a doctor's office visit. When offered a choice between an office-visit with a $100 co-pay and a $59 telemedicine visit, they will overwhelmingly choose the telemedicine visit. But what if a telemedicine visit or a cheaper alternative isn't offered? These patients may rely on treating themselves with advice from random Internet sites. Alternatively, they may not do anything and continue to live with their condition. Delaying a diagnosis of serious health condition and not starting appropriate timely treatment will result in higher healthcare costs when this patient ends up going to the emergency room. The bottom line is that we have a large and growing segment made up of price-sensitive individuals looking for more affordable healthcare, and telemedicine is a good solution.

On the physician side, we're seeing an increase in risk-based reimbursement contracts and reimbursement cuts for traditional services. The risk-based reimbursement approach is also known under some other names, such as risk-sharing agreement, accountable care organizations (ACOs), and bundled payments.

The overall goal of these approaches is to reward physicians for improvements in health outcomes and costs. The reimbursements are tied to quality metrics for the provider's entire population of patients. The idea is that medical providers are no longer heavily encouraged to conduct expensive tests and procedures, and instead shift their focus to preventing health issues and catching problems early.

In the risk-based reimbursement model, telemedicine is becoming a powerful tool. Telemedicine visits are cheaper and save physician time. They are more convenient for patients, which means that many patients are more likely to do a virtual telemedicine follow-up rather than show up in-person at the office. Some physicians can offer **two or more** convenient virtual follow-ups for their patients at the same cost to the patient as a **single** in-person visit.

Telemedicine is also receiving a legal push. Traditionally, government policies encouraged telemedicine only in rural clinics and for special situations. Now, many US states are putting in place telemedicine-favorable legislation for a wide array of conditions and use cases. In many states, medical boards are allowing physicians to see any new and existing patients with the help of telemedicine. In addition, many insurance companies have already been reimbursing telemedicine visits. We see new pieces of legislation addressing telemedicine every few months. We expect this trend to continue until all the U.S. states have fully embraced telemedicine.

The last major driving force in the wide adoption of telemedicine is technological -- the recent mass conversion to electronic medical records (EMRs) has paved the way for adoption of additional technologies. In early-to-mid 2000s, most private practices had separate physical rooms where all patient records were kept. Often, paper records weren't readily available, even at the physician's office, because they were kept at a remote record storage location. Medical treatment had to be done in the office. Physicians couldn't even take the records home due to HIPAA patient privacy guidelines. With the switch to EMR, physicians are now able to access records from anywhere with a secure Internet connection. And, even though the fax machine is still a staple of most medical offices, physicians everywhere became more and more comfortable using digital records, receiving labs, and sharing clinical data in digital formats.

In addition, today's EMRs allow for back and forth data transfer between other systems. This means medical providers using telemedicine platforms are able to exchange data with EMRs, other providers, and laboratory and radiology establishments. This leads to a seamless experience where patient data is instantly available and synchronized among multiple systems, saving time and money for physicians.

Definition of Telehealth

Before we go on, let's clear something up about telehealth. In some contexts, telemedicine is used specifically to refer to providing medical care, while telehealth includes telemedicine as well as additional non-clinical remote healthcare services such as education, technical support, and administration. In this book, we take the same stand as the American Telemedicine Association, that telemedicine and telehealth are effectively synonyms. [2] We will use them interchangeably, just like the words medicine and health (without the *tele-* prefix) are often used to mean the same thing when speaking about healthcare delivery. Another synonym for telemedicine that is occasionally used is *e-health*. By grouping telehealth and telemedicine together, we're expanding the definition of telemedicine. In this book we will largely focus on how modern technologies are used to deliver clinical services and exchange patient data.

The Brand New World of Telemedicine and Telehealth

Telemedicine is about connecting physicians and connecting patients. Fundamentally, it is about connecting people and sharing information with each other. This information may be pictures, text, lab results, or biological measurements.

In recent history, telemedicine wasn't always used to share information between physicians and patients. Although the patient was usually nearby, telemedicine was typically used to share information between a physician and another medical professional working with the patient. The use case was the following.

The physician was located in a central facility, such as a city hospital, while the medical professional sending the data was located in a remote location, such as a small rural clinic, a ship, a remote science station, etc. The medical professional sending data was the telepresenter – they used hardware specifically designed for telemedicine to transmit, or present, the medical information back to the physician. Yes, the patient was often there as well, but they weren't typically allowed to handle the equipment. The equipment was bulky, with lots of switches and options, and looked similar to other medical equipment one might see in a medical facility. The equipment was placed on a stand with wheels so it can be easily moved around. This telemedicine stand came with one or more cameras as well as special stethoscopes, blood pressure monitors, and other devices. These add-on devices were specifically designed or modified for transmitting data. The telepresenter, most often a nurse or a medical technician, had to be specially trained to use the equipment. Meanwhile, on the other end of the line, the physician received the clinical data using special equipment as well. And the information was sometimes sent using a special data protocol using a dedicated communication channel. This type of setup is what we refer to as *Telemedicine 1.0.*

Today, this type of telemedicine 1.0 setup is becoming less and less necessary. Majority of people in the US have a computer or a mobile device capable of taking and transmitting real-time video or high quality photos. Many modern clinical measurement instruments such as blood pressure monitors, digital stethoscopes, and ECG monitors are capable of transmitting data directly to the clinic's computer or the clinic's IT system. Equipment specifically designed for telemedicine is no longer absolutely necessary. In addition, patients are able to purchase affordable FDA-approved clinical measurement devices for use in their own home. Patients are becoming tech savvy and many are comfortable with figuring out these new high tech devices. Medical device manufacturers themselves see direct-to-consumer demand and, hence, are putting increased focus on ergonomic design and ease of use.

Today, using their own computing device and a few measurement devices purchased at the store, patients are able to effectively recreate the clinic's telemedicine setup in their own home. This growth in giving the patients and their physicians the capability to easily communicate directly with each other is what we refer to as *Telemedicine 2.0.* The "2.0" suffix typically refers to applications running on Web 2.0 technologies, characterized by their collaboration, usability, interoperation, and openness features. We adopt this moniker in this book. It is already frequently used in healthcare, with common terms such as Health 2.0 or Medicine 2.0. [3]

Here are a few examples of how telemedicine 2.0 can connect people:

- Telediagnosis – connect physician with patient
- Telepresence – connect physician, optional telepresenter, and patient
- Teleconsult – connect physician with another physician
- Telemonitoring – connect physician or nurse with patient
- Telesurgery – connect surgeon with patient during surgery

Telediagnosis, connecting physician directly with patient, is the biggest growing use case of telemedicine, and the one most of this book will focus on. Using telemedicine 1.0 technologies, the patient had to go through an intermediary, called telepresenter, in order to connect to a physician. Nowadays, using secure communication channels, patients regularly use their mobile phones, tablets, and laptops to send clinical information to their physician and get back an assessment, prescription, and a treatment plan. In this book, we mostly refer to telediagnosis as telemedicine virtual visits, or simply virtual visits.

Telepresence is the same use case as the traditional telemedicine 1.0 approach. However, due to advances in technology, this use case has grown in the number of situations it is used. Many paramedics, as telepresenters, now regularly use telemedicine to transfer video and patient vitals in real-time back to the physicians in the hospital. Using this information, the emergency care team instructs the paramedic and prepares before the patient arrival in order to provide care as quickly as possible. Also, instead of the traditional bulky telemedicine cart, today's telepresenters can use wireless digital stethoscopes, ultrasounds, and other instruments that send clinical data through their computer back to the physician. This means telepresenters don't need to be at the clinic to establish a connection, and this link can be done from the patient's home, an elderly care facility, a prison, or in any situation where the patient cannot travel. Today's physician, meanwhile, uses their day-to-day laptop or tablet to review the results. The physician can be located anywhere with an Internet connection.

Teleconsult, connecting physician with another physician, is a use case that we expect will grow tremendously in the next several years. An example situation is the following. A patient visits their primary care medical provider, and the provider, during the exam, finds a skin growth on the patient's leg. A consult with a dermatologist is needed. Normally, the medical provider would simply give one or more dermatologist names to the patient. Then, it would be the patient's responsibility to call the dermatology practice, schedule an appointment, and go in for a specialist office visit. Not to mention that many specialists may not have office visit openings for several weeks or even months. For example, the average wait time to see a dermatologist in Boston is 72 days. [4]

With a teleconsult, the primary care medical provider or their nurse would take proper photos of the patient's skin growth and send off the pictures along with patient's necessary medical information to the consulting dermatologists. The diagnosis could then be delivered directly to the patient or via the patient's primary medical provider. The patient or patient's insurance would be charged for the consult, and, if both the primary care and specialist physicians were employees of the same health system, the revenue would be shared between them. Although we give an example of a teleconsult arising from an in-person visit, a teleconsult can arise from telediagnosis as well.

The telemedicine consult may either be real time or asynchronous, where the information can be sent for later retrieval and review. Such consults save time and money, making care delivery more efficient for both patients and specialists. And primary care physicians aren't the only ones who could use teleconsults. Consults are frequently done between two specialists, or between a specialist and a sub-specialist. For example, a dermatologist may send a teleconsult case to a Mohs surgeon.

Telemonitoring is another growing application of telehealth. In many medical situations, such as postoperative recovery, the patient's vitals and other biological signs must be monitored in order to catch potential complications. For example, patient's weight must be monitored for fluid retention after heart surgery. By using wearable sensors, home measurement devices, and software to transmit the data back to the medical team, the patient may be sent home to recover much earlier than before. In addition, with the monitoring in place, the patient may not need to come into the office for post-surgery follow-ups. Telemonitoring is also being used for chronic conditions such as diabetes, heart disease, and mental illness.

Telesurgery is an exciting technology that has seen tremendous growth. Its poster child is the da Vinci Surgical System, which gives better visibility and control to one or more surgeons during a surgical procedure. The surgeons are often on-site with the patient, and simply located in an adjoining room. Additional less expensive telesurgery systems are rumored to be coming to the market in the near future. This book will not focus on telesurgery, as, at this point in time, the robotic surgery technology is very specialized and not readily accessible to many medical providers and patients.

The overall plan for this book is the following. First, we'll give a brief overview of the history of telemedicine. Next, we'll break up telemedicine into three major categories and discuss each in detail, including the benefits, challenges, and advice for implementing telemedicine deployments. Three major categories are store-and-forward telemedicine, real-time telemedicine, and remote patient monitoring. Then, we'll discuss a couple specific topics that medical practices need to be aware of when considering telemedicine, such as selecting a technology vendor and data security. Finally, we'll take a look at the future of telemedicine -- what's in store for Telemedicine 3.0 and beyond.

History of Telemedicine

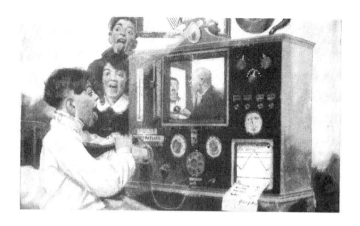

Telemedicine, you might be surprised to learn, was practiced in ancient times. That's because the history of telemedicine closely parallels the history of communication and information technologies. The key technical feature of telemedicine is being able to communicate medical data over a distance, and long distance communication methods existed throughout human history.

Some forms of medical information can be communicated over distance just as easily as any other verbal information. (Or, depending on your outlook and the age of the technology involved, they can be communicated with the same level of difficulty.) In the past, information that a new sovereign was crowned could be sent over the same long-distance communication medium as a warning about a dangerous disease outbreak. Here are a couple additional telemedicine examples that only require verbal communication:

- Identification, or diagnosis, of a specific medical condition based on a verbal description of the symptoms
- Prescription for the patient regarding what to eat and drink

In this chapter, we walk through telemedicine history until the present time. In the spirit of covering all of human history, we start in prehistoric times, before there was telemedicine.

Hunter-gatherer Telecommunication

Before the advent or agriculture, humans lived in hunter-gatherer communities. There are many hypotheses regarding the hunter-gatherer lifestyle. Here, we present our best understanding of this time period.

By their nature, hunter-gatherer communities were tightly-nit where everyone knew each other. Since permanent settlements didn't exist, the members of the community had to be fit enough to travel several days from one foraging place to another.

Many hunter-gatherer tribes had shamans, who, along with their religious responsibilities, were also *responsible* for medical care. Although, as you probably agree, the standards for quality of care were quite different back then, the tribe shaman was the go-to person when someone was ill. Depending on the tribe culture, some new shamans were trained through the apprentice system, while other shamans inherited their position, with the medical treatment methods and secrets being kept in one family's bloodline.

Since all members of the tribe were mobile and, generally speaking, together in one place, hunter-gatherers had little need for long distance communication. The default long distance communication technology, if we can even call it that, was the human messenger. Example uses for human messengers were:

- Sending messages between multiple tribes
- Sending an early messenger back from a successful hunt
- Coordination between multiple groups of a raiding party

No definitive evidence exists on the usage of telemedicine in hunter-gatherer societies. Still, we speculate that, in rare cases, shamans may have used human messengers to deliver medicine to the patient, or to exchange information and supplies with shamans in neighboring tribes.

Ancient Telemedicine

Let's fast-forward to the times of ancient Greece and Rome, around 500 BCE. By this point in human history, humans have mastered agriculture and lived in multiple nearby villages or towns. Communication between towns was common. Human messengers, of course, could still be used to transfer medical advice or medicine. Moreover, additional methods of long distance communication became widely adopted.

The major driver for improvements in long distance communication was the military. Cities needed to know as quickly as possible whether a foreign army was approaching, and be able to coordinate their own forces from a distance. Any other communication needs, medical or otherwise, were lower priority. Several widely used communication mediums included:

- Fires
- Smoke signals
- Light reflection beacons
- Drums
- Horns

Around the same historical time, we have evidence that some of these communication mediums, specifically smoke signals and light reflection, were used to communicate medical information. Specifically, long distance communication methods were used to signal the outbreaks of plagues and to notify about health events such as births or deaths. In North America, just like in ancient Greece, American Indian tribes also used smoke signals to relay medical calamities and health events. [5]

Early Telemedicine

The history of modern telemedicine, as we know it, was kicked off by the inventions of the electrical telegraph and the telephone. Although other inventions, such as flag semaphores and light telegraph, came onto the scene earlier, they were primarily used for military and naval communication. Before the telegraph and telephone, communication inventions did not expand the scope of telemedicine beyond ancient times. One exception is mail, another popular long-distance communication medium. Mail was used for medical communication. However, from a technological perspective, mail can be considered simply an extension of the human messenger.

The telegraph and telephone brought long distance communication into the mainstream, where almost anyone could send a telegraph message or make a phone call. Telegraph was still a special-use technology -- few individuals installed telegraphs in their homes due to the special training required to operate the telegraph, as well as due to the lack of a sufficient network of other telegraph receivers. Nevertheless, thanks to the communication speed of the telegraph, this technology was adopted for telemedicine in military situations. During the U.S. Civil War, telegraph was used for ordering medical supplies as well as communicating deaths and injuries on the battlefield. It seems likely that telegraph was also used for medical consultations. [6]

With the telephone, the era of the connected world arrived. Major city hospitals and doctor offices installed telephones. Within a few years, many city residents also had telephones in their homes. All of a sudden physicians could talk over the telephone to their patients and give medical advice directly. In addition, medical providers could speak over the phone to other physicians in order to consult or exchange information.

All of us, children of the modern world, take the telephone for granted. We've seen and used telephones from our childhood. Many people do not consciously consider the use of telephone as a telemedicine application. Patients don't consider it out of the ordinary when they discuss their blood test results or treatment recommendations with a nurse over the phone.

In fact, the use of the telephone is on the decline. [7] Many patients and physicians now prefer other asynchronous communication methods, such as secure text messages or emails via patient portals, which are more convenient. Still, the fact remains that the telephone was the foundation for many later communication and telemedicine technologies.

Through the 1900s, the overall usage of the telephone grew as the telephone network was enhanced with higher quality signals, telephone numbers, and other features. In 1968, 9-1-1 became the official emergency telephone number in the United States. The number could be used to report a fire, get the police, or a medical emergency. Previously, people using the telephone had to get the operator to forward their call to the right department (police, fire station, or hospital), or to know the specific number to dial. From a telemedicine perspective, 9-1-1 provided a consistent and faster access to emergency medical care.

Telefax, although invented before the telephone (and known as *electric printing telegraph*), did not gain significant traction until fax devices began to use the already existing telephone infrastructure and telephone numbers for transmissions. Shortly afterward, medical professionals began to use faxes en masse to transmit medical records. [8]

Rise of Telemedicine 1.0

The first idea of telemedicine as we know it today appeared in the April 1924 issue of *Radio News* magazine. [9] The magazine depicted using television and microphone for a patient to communicate with a doctor, including use of heartbeat and temperature indicators. The concept was an imagination of the future, as U.S. residents did not yet have televisions in their homes, and radio adoption was just gaining steam.

Proposals to transmit stethoscope readings and other instrument data over existing communication channels (telephone, radio, etc.) have been made in the first half of the 1900s. However, none of these one-off experiments picked up any traction.

The first uses of telemedicine to transmit video, images, and complex medical data occurred in the late 1950s and early 1960s. In 1959, the University of Nebraska used interactive telemedicine to transmit neurological examinations, which is widely considered the first case of a real-time video telemedicine consultation. Other programs followed, often implemented in an academic setting, which focused on transmission of medical data such as fluoroscopy images, x-rays, stethoscope sound, and electrocardiograms (ECGs). The main motivations of these early projects were:

- Providing access to healthcare in rural areas
- Urban medical emergency situations

A major break for the progress of telemedicine came in the 1960s when several partners, including the National Aeronautics and Space Administration (NASA), Lockheed Corporation, and U.S. Indian Health Service, joined together to work on STARPAHC project. STARPAHC stands for Space Technology Applied to Rural Papago Advanced Healthcare. The project provided telemedicine access to an American Indian reservation using the same technologies intended for astronauts on space missions.

Many additional grant and government-supported telemedicine initiatives followed, including:

- Providing medical care in a war zone
- Providing medical care to remote scientific stations in Arctic and Antarctic
- Providing medical care to correctional facilities without transporting inmates to the hospital
- Digital transmission of radiology images

Radiology was the first medical specialty to fully embrace telemedicine systems. With the help from grant-sponsored projects, which proved the reliability and efficiency of telemedicine, the medical community gained confidence in teleradiology. In 1980s some radiologists began to use teleradiology systems to receive images for telemedicine consultations.

In almost all of the early deployments of telemedicine, the telemedicine projects were large undertakings requiring considerable staff and organizational changes. Early telemedicine implementations used custom hardware and software equipment, often specifically created for the specific use case. The equipment was bulky and required specially trained personnel. This means the average patient did not directly interact with telemedicine technologies. Instead a telepresenter handled the equipment and interacted with the patient. Due to the advancement of technology and other factors, few early projects survived longer than 20 years in their original forms.

We use the term *Telemedicine 1.0* to refer to these early types of telemedicine deployments. Specifically, these projects are characterized by the following:

- Custom, bulky hardware specifically created for telemedicine

- Designed for specific use cases, such as psychiatry consults in ER
- Expensive
- Requiring specially trained telepresenters

Telemedicine and the Internet

The rise of the Internet in the 1990s also brought with it the information explosion. The Internet protocols allowed support for practically all information and traffic needed for telemedicine, including:

- Patient education (text, images, video)
- Medical images such as x-rays and scans (using DICOM image standards)
- Real-time audio and video consultation
- Vital signs and other body measurements (ECG, temperature, etc.)

Globalization, content publishing, consumer demand, and other factors outside of healthcare drove Internet growth. This growth meant that considerable funds and engineering efforts went into Internet infrastructure improvements, including:

- Communication speeds (bandwidth and latency)
- Information storage (databases, object-store for large files such as images and video)

- Availability – many web services employ back up servers, and even dynamically start up additional servers if traffic increases
- Standard formats for data transmission (MP4, PNG, etc.)
- Security (encryption, password protection, access levels, etc.)
- Application development -- new programming languages (JavaScript), frameworks, and open-source software (Apache)
- The Cloud – using virtual servers hosted by an infrastructure provider such as Amazon Web Services (AWS)
- Digitizing information (digital cameras, scanners, etc.)

The above communication infrastructure improvements had a positive impact on healthcare and telemedicine. All of a sudden it was easier and cheaper than ever to build a healthcare software application for exchanging and storing clinical data, using the existing tools and frameworks for web applications.

The e-health floodgates opened with the transition to electronic medical records (EMRs), boosted by U.S. government incentives. Most of today's EMR vendors employ the Internet in order to provide access to medical information for medical providers and patients. Patient portals have become common, where patients can look up their lab results or send a secure message to their physician.

Both medical providers and patients are becoming more and more technology savvy. The use of the Internet is commonplace in healthcare -- it is surprising to hear of a private practice without a web site. Many practices are trying to leverage the Internet further by engaging existing and potential new patients through social media outlets such as Facebook, Twitter and Google+. Some even reach out to their patients and encourage them to post reviews on Yelp and other review sites.

Patients, meanwhile, have access to tons of medical information online. Many patients research their symptoms using medical knowledge storehouses such as WebMD before coming to see their physician. Of course, one issue with getting information from public sources on the Internet is reliability – some online articles from questionable sources may mislead or confuse patients.

Today, the Internet is firmly established in day-to-day life. The majority of U.S. adults own a mobile device capable of accessing the Internet, such as a smart phone or tablet. Many rely on these devices as their primary entry point for the online world.

The ubiquity of the Internet, the ready access to Internet-enabled computing devices, and the technical savvy of the U.S. population are important factors in the ongoing *Telemedicine 2.0* transition. As mentioned in the introduction, the "2.0" suffix typically refers to applications running on Web 2.0 technologies. We adopt this moniker in this book. Telemedicine 2.0 is characterized as:

- Using existing computing device belonging to patient or physician
- Communicating over the Internet and using standard web infrastructure
- Using inexpensive off-the shelf equipment for gathering clinical data
- Easy to use -- can be used directly by patient or physician without special training

Some of the affordable measurement devices that are commonly used with telemedicine include, but are not limited to:

- Smartphone cameras
- Digital stethoscopes
- Ophthalmoscopes (for eye exams)
- Otoscopes (for ear exams)
- Vital sign monitoring devices
- Wearable biosensors

Telemedicine has now fully embraced the Internet communication medium. Many private practices and healthcare systems are in the process of becoming **hybrid healthcare providers** – allowing patients to see their medical provider either through telemedicine or in-person. We take a deeper look at the categories and types of Telemedicine 2.0 use cases in the next chapter.

Categories of Telemedicine 2.0

Telemedicine, the remote treatment of patients, is a broad concept that can't be definitively demonstrated by a single app or a monolithic piece of technology. It is a general concept of medical care delivery that has many approaches. Perhaps you've heard terms such as virtual visits, online appointments, and e-visits. Yes, these terms do refer to telemedicine, but they do so in the most general sense. They refer to replacing or augmenting a patient's office visit with one that is done remotely. Let's dig a little deeper into the types of telemedicine, as well as the uses, benefits, and drawbacks of each type.

When experts and academics talk about telemedicine, they break it up into categories. We'll do the same here in order to put a frame around which additional understanding can be built. Not all telemedicine companies offer all categories of telemedicine, not all categories are appropriate for every medical situation, and not all physicians are comfortable using every type of telemedicine. Telemedicine is not something that's completely unknown. In today's high tech world, the fact is that you're likely already using telemedicine even if you did not realize it.

The main categories of telemedicine are:

- Store-and-forward, also known as asynchronous
- Real-time, also known as live or interactive
- Remote Monitoring

In future chapters, we will go into detail for each category. In this chapter, we'll do a brief overview on each one to give the overall picture of today's telemedicine.

Store-and-forward telemedicine is asynchronous. To help understand that, let's use an analogy.

Almost everyone is familiar with email. It is an asynchronous communication technology. You send a message to someone. The recipient reviews the message some time later. While they're reviewing your message, you could be sleeping or browsing your favorite social media site, just to pick some examples. Of course, you could also be incessantly clicking the mailbox refresh button. Regardless of what you're doing, the point is that it's up to you – you don't need to always *be there* for the conversation to move forward. The recipient can spend as much time as they need on reviewing your message. Then, they carefully, or maybe not so carefully, draft a response and send their message back to you.

So, just like email, store-and-forward telemedicine does not require the physician and patient to *be there* at the same time. The patient sends images, medical history, and other necessary clinical information to the physician. Then, at a later time, the physician reviews the patient data, creates an assessment and plan, and sends back a response.

Let's give a real-life scenario. Suppose you wake up and notice a new rash on your leg that you can't seem to stop scratching. You have an important early meeting with your boss at work. So, you don't have time to think, much less deal with this medical issue. So, despite your rash, you rush off to the office. No pun intended.

After your meeting, you have ten minutes to spare. Normally, you would not do anything about your rash and hope it goes away. Or, if your spouse has been expounding recently about the importance of taking care of your health, you would schedule a visit with your dermatologist. You'd call the clinic and be told that there is a very long wait until the next opening. What a pain! It's almost like the stars are aligned against you getting medical care.

But now you know there is a better option. You sneak off to the bathroom. Using store-and-forward telemedicine software that your dermatologist's friendly medical assistant told you about, you take several pictures of the rash on your leg. Next, you send the photos as well as accompanying details to your dermatologist.

Later that day, between patient appointments, your physician takes 2 minutes to review your details and sends a prescription for an anti-itch cream to your pharmacy. You pick up the prescription on your way home from work. You apply the cream as directed, and feel better within hours.

Although store-and-forward telemedicine may sound new and exotic, you may in fact already be using it. Many practices have patient portals that patients can use to send messages to their physicians. Patients use these portals to send questions or request medications. That, by definition, is store-and-forward asynchronous telemedicine. And yes, physicians can (and some do) change money, often reimbursable by insurance, for these interactions when they provide medical advice.

The next major telemedicine category is **the real-time, interactive, or live telemedicine**. It is the category that most people think of when telemedicine is mentioned. Just like the name implies, patient and physician interact in real-time, such as through a phone conversation or a Skype-like live video encounter. Such interactions can be scheduled ahead of time, or occur spontaneously if both parties happen to be available.

So, when you're speaking to your physician over the phone, your conversation can be categorized as a real-time telemedicine visit. And yes, physicians can be reimbursed by insurance for such interactions as well. The question of when and whether to charge the patient is an important challenge to be covered in following chapters.

The last telemedicine category is **remote monitoring**. This category largely deals with biosensors that can be used to monitor patient's specific biological signs. Currently, remote monitoring is being used primarily for chronic diseases or specific medical conditions such as recovery from surgery.

Two representative examples of remote monitoring are glucose monitoring for diabetes and implantable devices for heart disease. Patients wear these devices every day. In turn, these devices regularly transmit data to the patient's physician. The data can be transmitted automatically from the devices or manually by the patient. For manual transmission, the patient simply writes down the numbers and either sends them electronically or brings the paper log to their next physician visit.

Recently, there has been an explosion of new biosensing wearables available on the market. In addition to existing off-the-shelf pedometer, heart rate, and sleep monitors, there are now wearable respiration, brain activity, oxygen level, blood pressure, and many other monitor and sensor types. [10]

At this point, many physicians do not recommend over-the-counter wearables for their patients to capture clinical data. The main reason is the perception that many wearables fail to provide medically significant, reliable, or sufficiently accurate data. There is a lack of sufficient medical research in wearable technology at this time. Nevertheless, such devices are being rapidly adopted by patients to improve their general health and well-being. Fitbit, the maker of the popular movement and activity monitor, has seen tremendous demand and filed for IPO (Initial Public Offering) in May of 2015. [11]

Mental health is another area that is rapidly adopting remote patient monitoring. Often, anomalies in patient's physical movement patterns, and even shifts in patient's mobile phone usage can act as a proxy for changes to their mental condition. These methods, in some cases, may signal early signs of depression and, thanks to remote monitoring alerts, allow medical providers and family members to quickly respond with interventions.

Now that we introduced the major telemedicine categories, we should also mention that physicians might choose to combine multiple categories into a compound approach. For example, a patient could be monitoring their weight and other biological signs, sending the physician reports using store-and-forward software, and occasionally talking to the physician in real-time over the phone. If you think that sounds complex, then you're correct. Physicians definitely need their patients to have some basic knowledge and experience with telemedicine 2.0 before throwing curveballs like this.

The fact that telemedicine has several approaches, and the fact that clinics and technology vendors often refer to them in generic terms such as *virtual visits*, can (and does) cause confusion for patients.

For example, one of our customer's patients was scheduled for a store-and-forward follow-up visit two weeks after the initial in-person appointment. Around the time of her follow-up, she contacted our 24/7 helpline and asked what time the visit would be. Her impression was that a virtual visit must be a real-time video visit – she did not understand that a medical virtual follow-up could be done asynchronously. Fortuitously, this patient was glad to learn that she was able to initiate her virtual medical appointment patient right away without waiting for the physician. When clinics are signing up their patients to use telemedicine, medical providers, staff, and software vendors should design a clear and simple approach to educate consumers to increase the understanding of telemedicine, thus increasing utilization of virtual visits.

Store-and-Forward (Asynchronous) Telemedicine

In this chapter we will cover store-and-forward telemedicine. Store-and-forward telemedicine is an asynchronous way to interact between doctor and patient. The approach is similar to email – the patient sends over their medical images and necessary clinical details, and physician reviews them at their convenience.

A Brief Word About Security

Now, you might wonder: if store-and-forward telemedicine is just like email, then why can't we simply use email to communicate with patients? That's because email is not secure and does not meet the security requirements of HIPAA (Health Insurance Portability and Accountability Act). HIPAA security is a complex topic, which we will cover in depth in a later chapter.

Suffice it to say that physicians cannot just use email and text messages to provide treatment or gather patient medical information. If you, as a patient, even wondered why your physician asks you to use a dedicated online system to either upload your medical information or read your clinical labs report, then at least part of that reason is due to security and patient privacy.

But wait, you may say that you went to your child's pediatrician, and she told you to "just text" her issues and pictures using standard unsecure MMS messages. Depending on the rules of your state's medical board, a physician may be allowed to use supplemental unsecure methods of communication such as email or text with their patient, but only if the patient explicitly authorized the use of such communication. [12] That said, the American Medical Association (AMA) guidelines generally advise against using unsecure or public connection to transmit patient data. [13] Violators may lose their medical license or be disciplined by their medical board. If that wasn't enough of a discouragement, a physician's medical malpractice insurance may explicitly forbid the use of unsecure communication, since it opens up another area of legal liability for medical providers. For all these reasons, we strongly recommend only using secure HIPAA compliant software for communicating with patients and transmitting patient data.

What is Store-and-Forward Telemedicine?

If we didn't scare you off already with that blurb about security, let's get back to the main subject of this chapter, which is the benefits and disadvantages of store-and-forward telemedicine.

Store-and-forward telemedicine is often compared and contrasted to real-time telemedicine. One popular impression is that real-time telemedicine uses video while store-and-forward does not. This is not strictly true -- store-and-forward technologies are able to use the same communication mediums, such as video and voice, as real-time telemedicine. In fact, from a technical perspective, store-and-forward uses many more mediums compared to real-time, including photos, medical images, forms, etc. The key difference between the two is that in contrast to real-time telemedicine, store-and-forward telemedicine does not require the medical provider and patient to be available at the same time.

Let's give a brief example. During a dermatology store-and-forward telemedicine visit for a skin rash, patient may do any or all of the following:

- Fill out a form
- Answer a customized questionnaire
- Take pictures of the problem area
- Record a video of the problem area while actively pinching the skin in order to give the physician an additional perspective

- Record a voice memo describing their medical history

That said, most store-and-forward telemedicine software solutions and usage models do not include video or voice component from patient to physician. The most likely reason is because video and voice recordings take longer for physicians to review than plain text, pictures, and raw data. Most often store-and-forward video and voice is used for communicating medical advice -- from medical provider to patient. One authentic example of store-and-forward video is patient discharge instructions. Patients leaving the hospital are required to receive often-lengthy written discharge instructions. By the time the patients get home, they may have forgotten certain specifics. Luckily, with asynchronous telemedicine, having the instructions available on video gets around this problem and potentially helps increase patient safety.

Teleradiology – The Store-and-Forward Poster Child

The medical specialty that has experienced a huge boom in store-and-forward telemedicine, starting with the rise of the Internet in 1990s, is radiology. Most radiologists today use modern store-and-forward telemedicine software to see cases from a remote location. Asynchronous telemedicine is also used when a general radiologists needs a consult from a sub-specialist, such as a pediatric radiologist. The significant shift of this specialty to the regular use of telemedicine software has resulted in major changes to the practice of radiology. The market for imaging procedures has been growing 15% annually despite only a modest growth of 2% in the number of radiologists. [14] Store-and-forward telemedicine is a major component of this growth -- telemedicine and other technologies have helped increase the productivity of individual radiologists, and allowed the industry growth to continue.

Another change in radiology has been the expectation, and even pressure, for 24/7 availability of radiology specialists. Physicians in emergency departments of many hospitals can order images in the middle of the night and send them to a radiologist for a turnaround of minutes or hours. This expectation of on-call availability has had a negative quality of life impact on radiologists. In response, firms have sprung up offering off-site teleradiology and on-call services. Such firms have radiologists on staff who hold medical licenses in multiple states. This allows a firm to maintain a large case volume by receiving cases from around the country. Radiologists work in shifts, which allows practices to significantly reduce or eliminate the needed on-call time for any individual radiologist.

Benefits of Store-and-Forward Telemedicine

Let's shift our discussion to the benefits of store-and-forward telemedicine. Some of the specific benefits and disadvantages that we'll discuss below also apply to real-time and remote monitoring telemedicine categories. We will cover these topics in detail in this chapter, and also briefly call them out in future chapters when discussing their relevance to real-time telemedicine or remote monitoring.

Main benefits of store-and-forward telemedicine include:

- Convenience and access to care
- Patient satisfaction
- Time savings for medical providers and patients
- Maximizing practice efficiency
- Attracting new patients and growing the market
- Reduced liability due to completely digital audit trail
- Easier physician education and consults
- Reduced physician overhead costs

Convenience and Access to Care

From a patient's perspective, convenience and access to care is one of the biggest benefits. By taking advantage of a virtual store-and-forward visit, patients minimize the interruption to their busy workday. We have spoken to several patients who regularly go to their physician for treatment of their chronic disease or specific condition. One example in dermatology is the treatment of severe acne with Isotretinoin (popularly known as Accutane). Regular monthly follow-ups are required for patients taking Accutane. Another example in dermatology is psoriasis, which is a chronic skin condition causing cells to build up rapidly on the surface of the skin, forming red patches. The patient schedules the visit on the phone, and often must wait on hold before even speaking to a scheduler. Then, the patient travels to the physician's office, waits in the waiting room, and waits in the exam room. After about 1-2 hours total waiting time, the patient sees their physician for a few minutes. The skin condition appears stable, the patient's prescription is renewed, and the patient drives back. These types of visits are good candidates for store-and-forward telemedicine – they are patients with an existing diagnosis that simply need monitoring via regular checkups. Of course, not all types of patients may be eligible, and it is up to the medical provider and the patient's preference whether to engage the virtual visit option.

Many patients are located in rural areas or otherwise underserved by physicians, such as West Texas. They must travel long distance to get to a physician's office, especially when seeing a specialist. For some patients, this means taking the day off work, which they may not be able to afford. Being able to see their physician virtually not only saves them time and frustration, but saves them travel and opportunity cost as well.

To take convenience a step further, asynchronous telemedicine visits don't have to be done during a workday at all. Patients can complete them during the weekend, in the evening, or at night. Just because the clinic hours are weekdays 9 am to 5 pm doesn't mean the patient treatment needs to be delayed.

Just as asynchronous telemedicine visits are more convenient for patients, they are also more convenient for medical providers. Physicians can review virtual patient visits in between in-person patient visits, during random openings in their schedule, such as due to cancellations or no-shows, or after clinic hours when their paid staff are off the clock.

Patient Satisfaction

Multiple studies have been published on patient satisfaction with telemedicine, and the general findings show that patients are satisfied with telemedicine. [15] [16] [17] Most patients are at least as satisfied with a telemedicine visit as they are with an in-person visit. Many patients actually prefer virtual visits instead of in-person visits.

Time Savings for Medical Providers and Patients

The short time needed to complete a store-and-forward visit is another advantage. As already mentioned above, for patients this benefit manifests mainly by eliminating the need to take time off work, and saving travel and wait time, compared the alternative of seeing the physician in person.

For physicians, speed and the associated saved time is one of the biggest, if not the biggest, benefits. While an in-person visit generally takes at least 10 minutes and could take 30 minutes or more, reviewing a store-and-forward visit takes as little as 2 minutes, based on our experience using an asynchronous platform. Even though the time is significantly less, it is still possible for physicians to provide high quality care over store-and-forward telemedicine. Part of the speed advantage for a physician comes from the fact that many top store-and-forward telemedicine solutions are optimized to help the medical provider detect the most common conditions for the given specialty. The way this is done is the following: the software-driven questionnaire asks the patient targeted questions, and, depending on the responses, the next questions are automatically selected to dig deeper into the patient's likely conditions. Thus, by setting up an intelligent questionnaire for the patient, the telemedicine system gathers the necessary clinical information. The physician sees all the relevant information in a single glance and is able to quickly make the assessment and treatment plan for the patient. The saved time for the physician comes from not having to ask the questions in real-time, and letting the software handle this largely repetitive task.

Some store-and-forward telemedicine systems allow physicians to customize the questionnaires and the information collected from patients. This allows the medical providers to fine tune the information gathered during a store-and-forward visit to exactly match the information they would have gathered during an equivalent in-person visit. This customization greatly reduces the common complaint about store-and-forward telemedicine that some patient information needed to make a diagnosis may be missing – the medical provider receives exactly what they asked for from the patient.

Let's take speed and saved time a step further. From a practice perspective, although reviewing occasional online visits provides tangible benefits, even more benefit can be accrued from batching. When a practice sees a significant number of patients as online store-and-forward visits, the physician, at their discretion, will only have to sit down once to review all of them as a single batch. For example, a medical provider can sit down for 30 minutes and review about 15 virtual visits, effectively doing a half-day of clinic work in half an hour. All of that can be accomplished with minimal to no medical staff involvement. In this example, we assume that most of these visits are routine, with little to no complexity.

Maximize Practice Efficiency

Speed and practice efficiency go hand in hand. Store-and-forward telemedicine is a great tool for schedule conflicts that can arise for patients and physicians. Frequent follow-up visits are ideal candidates for telemedicine. These types of visits are generally the lowest reimbursed visits by insurance. By shifting these types of visits onto a telemedicine platform, physicians free up their clinic schedule for more procedures, new patient consults, and other urgent cases – they gain additional time for their complex patients.

Another important consideration for running an efficient practice is dealing with

cancellations and no-shows – a patient is scheduled for an in-person follow-up, but they either cancel or don't show up to their appointment. Some clinics may supplement their in-person visits with telemedicine visits for the primary purpose of reducing their in-person no-show rates, smoothing out their schedule, and providing alternatives to their schedule-challenged patients. Doing this may not only increase patient satisfaction across the board, but may also bring in additional revenue from virtual patient visits, which would otherwise be lost. Seeing patients quickly and more efficiently provides an additional community health benefit – patients requiring medical care receive treatment when they need it, rather than prolonging suffering from delaying treatment.

Let's list several situations where a store-and-forward telemedicine replacement comes in handy. First, let's address the no-show case. Depending on the practice and the types of patients, some clinics experience over 50% no-show rate. [18] The high no-show rates and the chaos that goes along with them are a major inconvenience for both physicians and patients. Sadly, or perhaps fortuitously, physicians often know which patients will likely miss their appointment based on the patient's previous appointment-keeping record and physician's personal experience with such patients. Hence, as a general guideline, medical providers could recommend a store-and-forward virtual follow-up visit to such schedule-challenged patients. Such strategy may ward off some but no all no-shows. When other in-person patients do not show up to their original appointment, clinics could also automatically send an invitation for those patients to complete a virtual visit that very same day. This will not only provide better care to the patient, but also recover some of physician's lost time and revenue. If the clinic's telemedicine solution doesn't support such an auto-schedule feature, then clinics should try and shift such patients to virtual visits when these patients call to reschedule – suggest to them a virtual follow-up instead of scheduling yet another in-person follow-up. In addition, when a patient does not show up or cancels office visit, it takes away from another patient who has been waiting to see a doctor for weeks.

As much as we'd like to think so, telemedicine isn't the only solution to reducing a clinic's no-show rates. Traditionally, to make up the no-shows, clinics employ several strategies. One strategy is to double book the clinic's appointments. If you, as a patient, ever had to wait in a clinic for several hours to see your physician, you may be experiencing one of those times when all of your doctor's patients actually showed up for their appointments. It's not a good situation for anyone -- patients don't like the wait times, while physicians are under pressure to provide quality care to more patients than they have time for.

Another no-show reducing strategy is to charge the patient a fee if they didn't show up for their scheduled appointment. This approach has several logistical challenges. Clinics must collect and store patient's credit card information, and ensure the cards are valid and not expired. When the patient's co-pay is very low or non-existent, patients may balk at this approach. With all that, the typical fee charged for a no-show will still not make up for the lost revenue of a real visit. Everyone wins if the patient shows up in the first place.

The third strategy, claimed by physicians to be used very rarely, is to "fire" the repeat offenders who don't show up or cancel office visits. By not showing up to appointments, patients are effectively not adhering to medical advice, which makes treating them even more challenging. When clinics "fire" a patient, they remove this patient from the clinic's patient panel and do not schedule any more appointments for that patient. It is an unfortunate fact that many medical providers will not see such "blacklist" patients. The practice must be fairly established to employ this strategy on a regular basis, and be prepared to handle potential backlash and bad reviews from some disgruntled patients on social media sites, such as Yelp. After all, patients may have financial issues, a legitimate emergency or other mitigating circumstance that prevented them from making it to the appointment.

The traditional no-show strategies listed above are not perfect since all of them may antagonize patients. Our suggestion is to use store-and-forward telemedicine to recover lost visits, and convert schedule-challenged patients to virtual-visits. Here are several recommendations for an efficient **hybrid practice** that uses both store-and-forward telemedicine and in-person visits:

1. Offer to schedule all eligible follow-up appointments as virtual visits.
2. When a patient no-shows for an appointment and they're eligible for a virtual visit, immediately send them an alert. The alert message should offer a virtual store-and-forward visit that very same day, as an alternative way to be seen by their physician.
3. When a patient calls to cancel their appointment, suggest a virtual visit instead (if appropriate).
4. This recommendation is for clinics that double book appointments. When the clinic is falling behind schedule, call remaining patients on the schedule and recommend a virtual visit instead, if appropriate. Patients may be delighted to switch, or at least be glad for the heads up.

Attract New Patients and Grow Your Market

Now, let's talk about attracting new patients. Even when people have medical issues, many of them either refuse or are somehow prevented from going to the doctor's office. They may be hoping the issue will go away; they may not have the time to go to the clinic or even to schedule a visit; they may be embarrassed to admit they have a problem; or they may have one of a myriad other reasons. Many clinics are now using store-and-forward telemedicine to attract new patients, including attracting the above-mentioned ones who wouldn't have gone to the doctor otherwise. Store-and-forward telemedicine allows patients to quickly see a doctor on their own schedule and in their own environment. Thus, by giving patients access to a new technology for receiving medical care, telemedicine allows physicians to grow their overall patient market. This contrasts with the traditional view where one practice gains a patient at the expense of another practice.

One example of a workflow for such clinics is the following. When a patient visits a clinic's web site, they are prompted to start a virtual visit, either with a pop-up, a message, or a button. If the patient agrees to start a virtual visit, they are taken into the store-and-forward telemedicine application. First, the patient must answer several screening questions such as state of residence, insurance coverage, etc. Then, the patient goes through the virtual visit flow – provides the information on their issue, uploads pictures, and enters their medical history. In the end, either insurance or the patient must pay for this virtual visit, with payments ranging from $0 to $150. Copay may vary and depend on how quickly a patient would like a response back from a doctor. The payment amount may depend on the clinic, the telemedicine vendor, the type of visit, or other factors. Free virtual visits are typically offered as part of a concierge service or comprehensive treatment package, like a set price for plastic surgery with all follow-up appointments included.

After the patient is done, the physician receives an alert that patient has submitted their appointment. The physician reviews the visit and has several choices.

- Provide the patient with an assessment and treatment plan. Send a prescription to the patient's pharmacy, if needed.
- Recommend the patient come in for an in-person visit for further evaluation.
- Provide the patient with a possible diagnosis, prescribe treatment, and schedule the patient for in-person follow-up visit as well.

Using patient-initiated visits allows clinics access to patients that they may not have seen otherwise, using this increasingly important healthcare delivery mode. Sometimes, not all physicians in the practice will be willing to offer store-and-forward telemedicine visits. In that case, the clinic web site should list which physicians are available for virtual visits, and which ones only see their patients in-person. Alternatively, instead of prompting the patient to start a virtual visit from the practice's front page, the patient can be prompted to start a virtual visit when they come to the individual physician profile pages. But this alternative approach may reduce the number of potential new patients starting visits since some patients may never visit individual physician pages.

Detailed Documentation

The next advantage of store-and-forward telemedicine is detailed documentation, potentially resulting in reduced liability for the physician, thanks to the digital audit trail. Since the entire interaction between the patient and physician is digital, all information that the patient enters and the physician reviews are stored on the telemedicine application servers. In addition, due to HIPAA audit requirements, to be covered in a later chapter, every data access and change by the patient, physician, and any other provider with access to patient data is logged, along with the time of the access. Thus, the entire virtual patient-physician interaction is transparent, tracked in detail, and there is little to no ambiguity in the information presented to the physician or to the patient.

In contrast, real-time telemedicine interactions over phone or video are rarely recorded, from our experience. They are not recorded because these real-time data streams consume lots of digital storage space, and because, except in a few corner cases, the real-time interactions are not needed for later review. The real-time visits are documented just like in-person visits, with notes and updates the medical record. In-person visits as well as real-time video and phone discussions may open up the physician-patient interactions to later interpretations that may not have actually occurred or were intended during the actual visit. From a litigation perspective, store-and-forward telemedicine eliminates the gray area of "he said she said". Patient's and physician's answers, comments, recommendations and treatment plan are clearly documented, avoiding having to assume who meant what.

Easier Physician Education and Consults

Having the entire patient visit digitally documented and stored in the cloud gives additional benefits to the medical community.

One such benefit is education. Medical students, residents, and mid-level providers can be given past real or simulated store-and-forward telemedicine cases in order to practice their skills. The professor or attending physician can then review their diagnosis and notes before final submission. This approach allows younger providers to quickly get a significant number of cases under their belt. They would see exactly the same information as a practicing physician would see. The content of the actual cases could be adjusted for a focused training, giving younger providers a steeper learning curve, resulting in a faster time-to-competency.

Another benefit of digitally stored telemedicine visits is easier and more convenient consultations. Since all the relevant medical data is already available, allowing a physician in another location to take a look at the data could be as easy as adding the consulting physician's account to the telemedicine system. This often happens when a generalist wants a second look from a specialist, or a specialist wants a second look from a sub-specialist, like a dermatologist consulting with a pediatric dermatologist.

Reduced Physician Overhead Costs

Last but not least, virtual visits significantly decrease overhead costs to physician practices. For in-person visits, many clinic employees are involved in facilitating the patient's visit before a physician sees the patient in the office. Typically, before physically seeing the physician, the patient will have contact with a telephone operator, a scheduler, a medical assistant and sometimes even a mid-level provider.

Challenges of Store-and-Forward Telemedicine

Now that we've covered the benefits of store-and-forward telemedicine, let's cover the other side of the coin. The challenges, disadvantages and risks include:

- New Technology
- Patient uneasiness
- Insufficient patient information
- Medical insurance coverage
- Malpractice insurance coverage
- Potential conflict with existing methods, such as on-call availability
- Time and money needed for training providers, office staff, and patients
- Integration with existing systems and workflows
- Cost

New Technology

Although telemedicine has been around for decades, it is still seen as a new technology. One reason is the rise of new Telemedicine 2.0 applications thanks to the speed of innovation in software and the continuous stream of new offerings on the market. In the past, traditional telemedicine has been used to send information between a rural clinic and a city hospital, improving access in underserved areas. Today's telemedicine is increasingly being used to connect patients and physicians directly, regardless where they live. This means that software and hardware vendors are increasingly relying on devices that patients already have, such as mobile phones and tablets. A patient can download an app or go to a mobile-friendly web site -- they are able to complete their virtual office visit using their existing device from anywhere in the world with an Internet connection.

In our opinion, another reason for the perceived *newness* is the increasing adoption of telemedicine in the last several years. Although, as mentioned above and in a preceding chapter, telemedicine has been around for a while, its use has been primarily in academic and military settings. Most physicians with established practices have never encountered it, and even some newer physicians have gone through academic programs and residencies without exposure to telemedicine. However, today's telemedicine companies are marketing telemedicine solutions to hospitals, private practices, and directly to consumers. And this exposure does make telemedicine *new* for these settings and care models.

The risks associated with the *newness* of telemedicine are the same risks associated with any new technology. One recent transition in Health IT has been the transition from paper records to electronic records. Over 50% of practices now use Electronic Medical Records (EMRs) or Electronic Health Records (EHRs) systems. [19] However, although these technologies have provided many benefits, many physicians and medical staff still view these systems as clunky and hard to use. [20] [21] Many clinics and hospitals have adopted these technologies practically kicking and screaming solely to meet the government Affordable Care Act (ACA) requirements. For many, it is often easier to stay with the status quo because the perceived risk of not changing is lower.

Some of the common *newness* concerns include:

- What exactly is it, and how will it impact my current level of service?
- Will it work? Is it going to do what the telemedicine provider claims it does?

- What if it breaks? What do I do when the Internet connection is down?
- How much time and effort will I have to spend to figure this thing out?
- I don't see my competitors using it. Why should I be an early adopter?

One of the reasons for writing this book is to dispel some of these concerns, and to provide education for both medical providers and patients regarding the care models, business models, and technologies behind telemedicine. To address the above questions – yes, telemedicine works and, in our opinion, provides tangible benefits for patients, physicians, and practice managers. At the same time, just as with any change, there is a learning curve.

Patient Uneasiness

We mentioned patient satisfaction as a benefit above, but we now mention patient uneasiness as a risk. You can't have it all. Some patients may approach store-and-forward visits with caution, and may choose to stick to in-person visits even if telemedicine visits are available. Some types of patients actually like going to the doctor – it's a break from work, they like spending some time with their physician and with medical staff, and travel time is not a big issue. It's possible that many of these patients probably have lots of free time and a very flexible schedule. Luckily, most of the patients who are either not interested or won't be satisfied with telemedicine simply will not choose a telemedicine visits if given a choice between an in-person and a virtual visit. These types of patients will self-select themselves out of being telemedicine users.

However, physicians and medical staff can also unintentionally lower patient satisfaction depending how effective and versed they are in using the telemedicine software. To ease such potential issues, below are a few important telemedicine software usage guidelines:

- Do NOT ignore patient virtual visits that need attention – try to review and respond to all virtual visits within 24 hours or, even better, on the day they are submitted
- Do provide adequate, detailed, and clearly written visit report to the patient
- Do NOT request all patients doing a virtual visit to come in for an in-person visit as well. Only request in-person visits for patients who cannot be adequately assessed with store-and-forward telemedicine.
- Do inform patients that they can always switch to an in-person visit if desired

Here is one more point to keep in mind. It's important to differentiate between patient satisfaction with telemedicine and patient satisfaction with their treatment plan. Sometimes patients are happy with store-and-forward telemedicine, but dissatisfied with their treatment plan.

Insufficient Patient Information

Have you ever been to a doctor and been asked to fill out the same form and answer the same questions that you already filled out on every single previous visit? And then you wondered if the clinic knows what they're doing, and why do they subject you to such torture? How many times must you list the same surgery you had when you were a teenager? One danger every physician faces is insufficient or missing patient information. If a patient forgets to mention a drug they are taking or a medical condition they have, their physician may prescribe a drug that will results in a dangerous drug interaction or worsen a medical condition.

One example is the following. A patient with a condition visits a specialist, but fails to mention the medication prescribed by their primary care provider that they're currently taking. The specialist prescribes them the same drug, but under a different brand name. Patient fills the prescription at a different pharmacy, and now takes both pills, without realizing that they are the same drug, just different brand names. This patient takes a double dose, increasing their risk of adverse health outcomes.

One way to mitigate this risk is to ask every patient to fill out their medical information every time, so as to better catch any changes or details that are prone to fall through the cracks. Of course, a better alternative would be for a patient to simply review, amend, and confirm their information instead. However, many practices may not be integrated or set up for such a workflow.

The convenience, speed, and user-friendliness of store-and-forward telemedicine software may make it easy for patients to accidentally skip or under-report their allergies, current medications, or medical history. Even if the patient skips reporting a medication, figuring that the physician already knows about it, this prescription information may actually be in a separate system, such as an EMR, or the physician may assume the patient is no longer taking that medication. Since store-and-forward telemedicine is not real time, going back and asking the patient to verify their medication is not an acceptable workaround, because it would take additional turnaround time, delay care, and may be an inconvenience for both the patient and the physician. On the other hand, asking patients questions such as "Are you sure you are not taking any medications?" may be viewed as an annoyance and result in lower patient satisfaction with the overall telemedicine visit. When it comes to missing patient information, the clinic's telemedicine software must support a flow that the physician is comfortable with. The ideal flow captures patient information as smoothly as possible, without disrupting efficiency.

Patient information may either be missing because the patient did not enter it, or patient information may be missing because it was not gathered. As we mentioned above when discussing the benefits of store-and-forward telemedicine, the top software solutions use intelligent questionnaires that are optimized to detect the most common medical conditions for a given specialty. Thus, in our opinion, the problem of not asking the patient the right questions during a store-and-forward telemedicine visit has been greatly mitigated, although risk still exists. Not gathering appropriate and necessary information may especially be a challenge for very rare conditions. Still, a certain number of patients will have rare conditions or rare complications. In those cases, lacking sufficient data, physician may need to see the patient in-person to assess the issue further. The exact percent of such cases largely depends on the specialty and the provider's patient mix.

There is also a potential benefit for patient information with telemedicine. Since many patients will be completing their virtual visits from home, they may have convenient access to their medications. This means if they don't remember the exact name of the medication that they are taking, they could simply go to their medicine cabinet and read the label on the medicine container.

Just as physicians may find the patient information insufficient, patients may likewise find the physician report and treatment plan insufficient. Patients may have questions and clarification requests after the telemedicine visit is complete. There are a couple approaches to help handle such patient questions. One approach is to encourage patients to call the clinic, and triage their questions. A medical assistant or nurse may be able to answer the question without getting the physician on the line. Another approach is to use a messaging feature common to many telemedicine applications, where patients can send messages to their physician. This approach is similar to email or patient portal messaging. Some telemedicine applications may limit the number of messages or the amount of time after the virtual visit when such messages can be sent. Since the patient or patient's insurance has already paid for the visit, this patient service offers no additional financial value for the clinic. Some physicians that we spoke with have voiced concern that some patients may abuse the follow-up messaging and support service. However, this approach is not significantly different from existing approaches, such as a clinic's on-call service or sending messages through a patient portal.

Medical Insurance Coverage

One of the most common questions we hear when speaking with potential customers and business partners is: "Is it covered by insurance?" The simple answer is: "Yes, in many cases." But, as with most things in healthcare, the answer is more complex.

State laws regarding insurance reimbursement and insurance coverage govern medical insurance. Most states now have telemedicine parity laws -- these laws dictate what types of telemedicine must be covered by insurance, and, in many cases, what the reimbursement rate should be for those visits. [22] The types of telemedicine covered include not only categories, such as store-and-forward versus asynchronous, but also care models, such as initial diagnosis versus follow-up for established diagnosis, as well. Furthermore, the laws may even have different rules for different specialties, with mental health being the primary example. For instance, laws may allow coverage of real-time video visits but not store-and-forward visits. Laws may allow coverage for follow-up care but not initial diagnosis, except for psychiatry visits. Laws may dictate that the insurance reimbursement rate must be the same for in-person visits as for telemedicine visits, or they may leave the exact reimbursement flexible. Yes, the insurance landscape is complex.

In addition to reimbursement and coverage, insurance companies themselves maintain separate divisions, often with separate insurance policies for each state. So if one insurance company reimburses store-and-forward telemedicine visits at one rate in one state, that is not necessarily the case for a different state. The state divisions are done by law, although many industry advocates we spoke with would like to change the law to allow insurance companies to operate across state lines. In addition, some insurance companies and self-insured organizations view telemedicine as a competitive advantage – a way to reduce healthcare costs and improve population health. One example is Home Depot. [23] Thus, regardless of state laws, these forward-looking entities may decide to always reimburse telemedicine. They may even offer telemedicine visits for free to their members, going beyond of their state's minimum requirements.

Thus, unless the clinic only accepts cash or telemedicine is explicitly not covered in their insurance contract, either the telemedicine vendor or practice has to deal with insurance. For virtual follow-ups, the clinic will already have the patient insurance information on file. In this case, assuming the telemedicine co-pay and payment schedule from the insurance company is already known, the medical staff can directly set the patient's co-pay when scheduling a telemedicine visit. For patient-initiated visits, the telemedicine software must gather the patient insurance information directly from the patient. Then, either the clinic staff or the telemedicine vendor must determine eligibility and submit the insurance claim.

We hope that, in the next several years, all insurance companies will provide eligibility and co-pay details in real-time – available instantaneously on request. This will benefit the patient because they will know up front how much a virtual visit will cost. Currently, if the insurance eligibility and co-pay details are not already known, the clinic must submit the claim before knowing the reimbursement amount and patient portion of the visit. Since in these cases the final charge may not be determined until days or weeks later, we recommend alerting the patient up front what their maximum financial responsibility could be.

Malpractice Insurance Coverage

Just like every state has different medical insurance policies, every state also has their own malpractice insurance policies and vendors. Unlike medical insurance laws, which are set by the state's legislature, malpractice insurance policies are influenced by the state's medical board. Malpractice insurance vendors may or may not cover all categories, care models, and specialties for telemedicine. Physician or telemedicine provider must check with the malpractice insurance company to see what they cover. The best telemedicine vendors will check with the top malpractice insurance providers in the state ahead of time and already have this information for potential customers. That said, even if malpractice insurance does not cover certain care models, a large enough practice could self-insure for telemedicine visits. In addition, some telemedicine providers are offering their own telemedicine malpractice insurance for physicians using their products. So far, telemedicine has had very few reported malpractice cases. As of 2015, Teladoc, a company that has been offering telemedicine visits for over 10 years, has not had a single malpractice insurance claim. [24]

Conflicts with Existing Patient Interaction Methods

Store-and-forward telemedicine provides new ways to interact with patients. Some of these ways may cause workflow conflicts with existing systems used by clinics. Many clinics have a doctor on-call after hours. If a patient has a question or concern, they can reach the on-call service when the practice is closed. (This, by the way, is a classic example of real-time telemedicine.) Some existing patients may use the on-call system to receive care for their new medical conditions, even though the on-call system is typically not intended for this use case. For example, in dermatology, a patient with a new poison ivy rash may call and get a prescription from the on-call physician. In most cases clinics do not charge for their on-call service. The physician, could, of course, at their discretion, ask the patient to come into the office instead of providing treatment directly over the telephone. However, in our experience, clinics typically do not have strict guidelines for their physicians regarding what can and cannot be done through their on-call service. They leave it up to the physician's discretion.

For clinics offering patient-initiated store-and-forward telemedicine, a patient coming to the clinic's web site may see two ways to receive non-emergency treatment after hours – call the on-call number or start an asynchronous telemedicine visit. (Here, for the on-call service, we're referring to clinic's existing patients. In our experience, clinics never provide on-call service to patients without a patient record or without a recent office visit, typically within the last 12-to-36 months, depending on the state and practice policies.) From a financial perspective, the medical practice will likely make more money if the patients use virtual store-and-forward telemedicine instead of using the on-call number. But, from a patient satisfaction standpoint, some patients may want the option to speak with a real live doctor when they want to. In addition, when patients know that on-call services are free, why would they ever agree to pay for a store-and-forward telemedicine visit? There is no easy solution here. Practices that have this issue will need to take steps to resolve this conflict so that they offer consistent service and pricing across all of their care models.

One option is to eliminate the traditional free telephone on-call service and only offer a paid and higher-value real-time video on-call service. Another option is to link these two types of services – require a patient to initiate a store-and-forward visit and enter all their clinical information before allowing them to speak with the on-call physician. This way the physician will already have all the information in front of them for a quick and efficient assessment. These alternative options must be considered in light of the relevant state laws.

Another patient interaction system commonly employed by clinics is a messaging system, typically via a patient portal. Patient can sign in to their patient portal and send a textual message to their physician. Technically, this type of interaction is considered store-and-forward telemedicine of the simplest type – simple messages that may or may not provide enough medically relevant information to the physician. From our experience, patients typically use this system for either simple follow-up questions regarding their previous visit or queries prior to their next visit. Since this type of simple messaging is open-ended and does not provide a structured flow, some patients seeking treatment of their existing or new condition may abuse it. On the other hand, structured store-and-forward questionnaires, where patients provide all relevant information to their physician, are more amenable to a paid model.

Staff Training

Today's clinics use a multitude of software products and services that include EMRs, payment and billing systems, scheduling systems, patient portals, and many others. A store-and-forward telemedicine system adds to the existing technological burden on physicians and medical staff. It is another system to learn, another set of username and passwords to maintain, and another system that patients will ask questions about. Just as with other systems in the clinic, providers and medical staff will need training.

Adopting telemedicine within an existing private practice or healthcare system is an organizational change – every member of organization, including physicians, mid-level providers, office managers, and medical staff, must be on board with the new workflows. All too often, telemedicine implementations fail because all the concerned parties did not buy into the idea, the organization does not take advantage of telemedicine in a disciplined way, and the process essentially falls apart. During staff training and ramp up, the telemedicine vendors and key medical personnel must communicate the benefits of telemedicine, including benefits to the patients and benefits to the clinic/healthcare system.

To achieve success with telemedicine, a multi-physician organization should also have a physician telemedicine champion. This physician should lead the way by:

- Using telemedicine whenever appropriate, and seeing a meaningful number patients using telemedicine.
- Communicating the benefits and reasons for using telemedicine to their peers.

- Working with the telemedicine vendor to develop best practices and flows for their organization.

If an organization adopts telemedicine without a physician champion, then this effectively means that the practice is relying on patients to be champions – to request telemedicine visits from physicians or to start the visits directly from the participating clinic's or the vendor's website. However, in order for patients to request a telemedicine visit, the patient should be informed and convinced that a virtual visit is the right path for them. Here we have a potential "chicken and the egg" dilemma – patients may be extremely willing and eager to use the clinic's telemedicine offering, but the clinic staff may not inform them that such a service is available because they did not get sufficient training or they believe patients do not prefer virtual visits. Our recommendation is that the practice provide plenty of information to the patients regarding the availability of telemedicine, as well as either directly answer the patients' questions or connect them with the vendor's support representative. For example, placing telemedicine brochures in the patient waiting area is a good start. We've seen plenty of patients, even older people in their 70s, embrace telemedicine visits when offered the choice. Otherwise, without either a strong physician drive or a patient education campaign, the practice may not reach a meaningful volume of telemedicine visits.

For private practices and organizations exploring using telemedicine, we recommend speaking to a medical provider who has been "through the trenches" – who implemented telemedicine in their practice and can elaborate regarding the everyday benefits and challenges of their implementation. The top telemedicine software vendors will have a staff or consulting physician available to help assess the risks, organizational changes, and specific next steps needed to achieve a successful transition to a hybrid practice. A hybrid practice is one that offers both in-person and telemedicine services.

Adding a store-and-forward telemedicine service to a clinic will not make life easier for medical staff initially. Although the system provides clear benefits to patients and physicians, the practice must take special care to communicate the benefits to the medical staff. The medical staff, along with the providers and the management team, must figure out how to fit the telemedicine service into existing systems and workflows. This includes knowing which system to use when, where the information is stored, and, if needed, how to transfer data from one system to another. There is also the traditional human reaction to resist changes in the status quo. In a couple private practices, we have seen pushback from the medical staff that prevented or delayed the transition to telemedicine. In addition, the transition period to telemedicine adds additional pressure on every person in the practice – they must not only continue performing their current duties but also ramp up and get ready to accept patient visits over telemedicine. The ramp up activities include attending training, updating or re-writing procedures, changing customer communication templates, and other tasks.

As part of the medical practice changeover process, employee job descriptions and expectations must be modified to be in line with the new business direction for the practice. For example, in addition to in-person patient satisfaction criteria, the practice will now need to consider the satisfaction of their online patients. During the initial transition process, it may be beneficial to offer incentives, such as gift cards, to everyone who achieves proficiency on the new system and workflows. In some cases, it may be necessary to define new compensation levels for the new and altered roles. We also recommend identifying or creating the role of a lead telemedicine staff member. This individual will have additional responsibilities, such as:

- Primary contact for scheduling telemedicine visits
- Ensuring that telemedicine visits are being processed quickly and efficiently

through the workflow, meeting patient
expectations for turnaround time
- First source of contact for patient
  questions and education
- Responsible for training new staff
  members joining the practice

Certain members of the clinic workforce may
never get on board with the new way of doing
business, and perhaps even try to actively
sabotage the effort. Although we hope this never
happens to you, such things do happen when
organizations undergo changes. Whether the
reason is because these individuals are afraid of
change, or due to some other personal reasons,
we will not try to speculate on the many reasons
why people resist organizational initiatives.
Organization's performance evaluation and other
employee incentive systems may need to be
adjusted to make sure everyone is on the same
page with telemedicine. If problems persist, and
resistant individuals are still causing havoc in the
critical part of the new workflow, these
employees should either be reassigned to
another role in the organization or replaced.

Integration with Existing Systems and Workflows

A new telemedicine system adds potential
duplication to existing systems in the clinic:

- Patients may have a virtual visit scheduled in the telemedicine system and an in-person visit scheduled in the regular system.
- Patients pay through the telemedicine system, and their payments must be reconciled with the regular payment system.
- Patient demographics are stored in both telemedicine system and EMR. If a patient updates their demographics in the telemedicine system, it must be synchronized with EMR.
- Patient allergies, medications, medical histories, and preferred pharmacies are stored in multiple systems.
- Physician could electronically send prescriptions from the telemedicine system or from their existing e-prescribe solution.
- After the patient completes a store-and-forward telemedicine visit, their encounter report and updated medications must be uploaded to the EMR so that the continuity of care requirement is met.

Although quite a few of the items and workflows listed above are potentially being duplicated, there is a solution here. The solution is to fully electronically integrate the telemedicine software with clinic's existing systems. By using HL7, FHIR, APIs, and other technical methods, a fully integrated telemedicine application will keep itself in sync with the clinic's existing systems. This two-way sync includes: pulling in patient demographics when needed, updating patient encounter notes and medication, updating billing, posting the virtual follow-up appointments in the scheduling system, etc. Hence, when the telemedicine solution is fully integrated into the clinic's workflows and systems, almost all friction points and ease-of-use concerns will be eliminated.

Transitioning from an in-person-only private practice to a hybrid practice that also accepts telemedicine patients requires changes in work processes and technology. Oftentimes, existing systems must be re-evaluated to see whether they still fit with this new way of doing business. Perhaps some existing systems, such as patient portal messaging or billing, do not fit into the new organizational workflow. In that case, these systems must either be upgraded/modified, replaced with another system, or, when functionality is already accomplished by other systems, completely eliminated. Elimination of systems occasionally happens in telemedicine adoption when certain types of visits and care models become primarily available via telemedicine without a readily available in-person alternative. For example, a practice with multiple locations may decide that at one of their locations certain types of visits, such as postsurgical follow-ups, will only be available over telemedicine. Any previous paper or electronic systems solely dedicated to those types of in-person appointments would be retired at that location. The patients would still have the option for an in-person follow-up, but they would need to travel to another location to see that provider.

Cost

The last item to consider for store-and-forward telemedicine is cost. Although telemedicine offers cost savings and improved practice efficiencies, it is not free. Also, the exact cost can vary depending on many factors, such as the size of medical content that is being stored for later retrieval. For example, high definition videos take up more digital space than mobile photos or text questionnaires. The telemedicine vendors often use one or a combination of the following pricing strategies:

- One time setup fee.
- A monthly or yearly ongoing fee. This fee may either be per provider or per clinic location, often with some minimum commitment.
- Revenue sharing – the telemedicine vendor either takes a percent or a set dollar amount of each telemedicine patient visit. Some telemedicine vendors

charge a percent of total collections for the provider.

In addition to the above-mentioned standard fees, the telemedicine vendors may charge for add-ons such as EMR integration, e-prescribing, white labeling, insurance eligibility lookup, and other features.

Telemedicine vendors typically do not publicize their prices because some of their customers have unique requirements that require special considerations. Some clinicians may view telemedicine as a way to make medical treatment affordable for their patients, while others position their virtual visit offering as a premium service. Some clinics may only want to use telemedicine for low-risk follow-up visits, while others see it as a marketing opportunity to attract new patients in the area.

The physician must consider the cost of the solution and whether it makes sense for their practice. For those clinicians who are not sure whether telemedicine is right for them or how often they will use it, the % of visit fee pricing model should make the most sense. This allows the physician to try telemedicine essentially cost and risk-free. And, as the clinic increases volume of their telemedicine visits, the revenue share approach may no longer make financial sense. When that happens, the practice should choose a recurring monthly fee option.

Ideally, to reach the maximum efficiencies offered by telemedicine, the physician should see several telemedicine patients per week. This will also make medical staff more familiar with the technology and the workflows, and will be more assuring to the patients. It is also a good idea to schedule all virtual follow-ups for the same weekday, if possible. This will allow the physician to review all such visits as a single batch.

Summary

In summary, store-and-forward telemedicine offers many benefits to patients and clinicians, including convenience, speed, and efficiency. However, clinics must also consider the potential challenges such as ramping up on new technology, checking on medical and malpractice insurance coverage, and integrating with existing systems and workflows.

Real-Time Telemedicine

In this chapter we will cover real-time, or interactive telemedicine. Just as the name implies, real-time telemedicine occurs when both parties are present on the line at the same time, or in real-time. The parties can be a patient and a medical provider, two or more medical professionals, a teacher and a medical student, or some combination of the above.

The most common mediums for real-time telemedicine are phone and video. Phone is the classic telemedicine communication medium that has been used for many decades. Real-time telemedicine over the phone is very common today, and many patients and physicians use it without realizing that it is categorized as telemedicine. Some everyday examples of telemedicine over the phone include:

- Patient speaking with on-call provider after clinic hours
- Nurse giving patient clinical lab results
- Medical provider following up with the patient after surgery
- Translator services used via phone to communicate with a patient who does not speak the same language as their provider

- Video relay interpreter service used to communicate with hearing impaired patients

Besides phone, the next most common medium for interactive telemedicine is video. Videoconferencing is what many people think of when the word telemedicine is mentioned. Part of that perception is due to the fact that, in the past half century, the *tele-* prefix has been increasingly used with things related to television.

In most of today's real-time video telemedicine encounters, the video is sent as encrypted traffic over a public or private Internet connection. A dedicated network link can be used, but such special infrastructure is rarely employed in newer telemedicine deployments.

Mental health is one of the largest growing segments for the adoption of real-time video telemedicine. A study with US Veterans Administration has found that PTSD patients receiving telemedicine counseling had significant improvement, in line with results expected from in-person visits. [25] Many psychiatrists are employing telemedicine to supplement their in-person visits. In fact, with the growing patient demand, it is now possible to have a 100% virtual mental health practice – virtual patient visits, as well as a virtual receptionist.

Radio is another medium used by real-time telemedicine, such as a two-way radio between paramedic and physician. It is considerably less common, and largely used in military and emergency telemedicine.

Text message is another popular communication method for the general public. The healthcare community is readily adopting texting to meet various communication needs. However, as mentioned in the beginning of the chapter on store-and-forward telemedicine, HIPAA security concerns require providers to use HIPAA-compliant messaging application.

Although a text message conversation often occurs when both parties are actively viewing and responding, this method of communication is commonly not considered real-time telemedicine. Text message applications, by their nature, generally do not require both parties to be online at the same time. The text message can be sent when the other party is not monitoring their text message application. This message can be asynchronously retrieved from the server or from the device minutes or hours later.

Benefits of Real-Time Telemedicine

Now, let's cover the benefits and challenges of real-time telemedicine. Some benefits and challenges of real-time telemedicine are similar to those for store-and-forward telemedicine. Since store-and-forward telemedicine was covered in the previous chapter, we will not repeat some of the specific details here, and only call out the differences and any information relevant to interactive telemedicine. The benefits of real-time telemedicine include:

- Great for patients
- Close match to in-person visit
- Increased practice efficiency
- Potentially better insurance coverage than store-and-forward
- Attracting new patients and growing the market

Great for Patients

Patient-centered benefit is one of the biggest drivers of real-time video telemedicine. Patients love the convenience of real-time telemedicine just as much as store-and-forward telemedicine. It minimizes interruptions to their day, eliminates travel, and reduces or eliminates waiting time. Patients are also satisfied with video visits just as much as with in-person visits. [17]

Close Match to In-Person Visit

Unlike store-and-forward telemedicine, interactive video visits are a much closer proxy for regular in-person visits. The key benefit is the presence of both parties, which allows for immediate back and forth between patient and medical provider to address questions and clarifications. Unlike store-and-forward telemedicine, where the physician and the patient may need to send several messages back and forth, the patient and the medical provider may get on the same page much faster when conversing in real-time. This also means that the physician may be able to give a more precise diagnosis to the patient, especially for rare conditions, during a real-time telemedicine visit because the provider is able to go further in depth and eliminate more potential causes of the condition. In contrast, during a store-and-forward visit, the physician is typically presented with information sufficient to diagnose the most common conditions of their specialty.

On the flip side, for many physicians their typical diagnosis is one out of the same familiar set of conditions. This means that during a real-time video visit the provider will typically ask the same questions and hear similar responses. The leading store-and-forward telemedicine software products are able to ask patients the same sequence of questions as a physician would ask, including asking the right follow-up questions. Nevertheless, the common patient and physician perceptions are that real-time telemedicine visits have the potential to accomplish more. Certain types of real-time visits, especially visits for rare conditions, will be able to be more productive than store-and-forward telemedicine. However, such visits constitute a small percent of patient volume, and many such appointments may require an additional in-person visit as well. In contrast, this is precisely what a physician reviewing an equivalent store-and-forward virtual appointment should recommend as well.

Increased Practice Efficiency

Real-time telemedicine can add some efficiency to the existing practice. That said, these efficiencies are a subset from those gained from store-and-forward telemedicine solutions. Whereas store-and-forward telemedicine allows the hybrid practice to shift some of their patients to virtual visits in order to free up in-person appointment slots for more severe medical cases, real-time telemedicine visits still take up approximately as much time as in-person appointments. This lack of any meaningful speed advantage from real-time visits does not allow the physician to see more patients in the same amount of time without expanding their clinic hours.

The practice efficiencies from real-time telemedicine largely come from administrative sources. While a physician is seeing patients virtually, they do not require to be present at, or to even have, an office. They do not need a receptionist, a waiting room, or exam rooms. If the physician does need an assistant for real-time telemedicine, their assistant may work remotely. Many physicians share offices with other providers. Some physicians have offices in multiple locations where they see patients. Accepting virtual video visits allows a physician or practice to reduce their office and staff overhead.

Since the interactive telemedicine visits do not need to be done in the office, physicians are free to adjust their clinic hours to be more in tune with their own schedule. Physicians can do the video telemedicine visits from their home early in the morning, in the evening, or on weekends. To give a more unusual example, suppose physician has clinic at two different locations in one day. If they hire a driver to take them from one location to the other, they can see real-time telemedicine visits while traveling.

Potentially Better Insurance Coverage Than Store-and-Forward

Today, insurance coverage is an advantage for real-time telemedicine when compared with store-and-forward telemedicine. The current medical insurance coverage laws and malpractice insurance coverage slightly favor real-time telemedicine over store-and-forward telemedicine. This means that in some states, depending on specialty and care models, patients that can be seen over real-time telemedicine cannot be seen via store-and-forward telemedicine. That said, this is a fast moving landscape that may have already changed after these words were written. Every month or two, we typically hear of new laws or policy changes favorably impacting telemedicine.

We fully expect regulations favorable to telemedicine to continue. In time, we expect real-time and store-and-forward telemedicine to be available across all specialties for both initial diagnosis and existing patient care models, including insurance coverage with $0 or low co-pays. Since real-time telemedicine visits generally take more time for physicians than store-and-forward visits due to the additional time conversing with patients, physicians generally demand higher reimbursements for real-time visits, on par with in-person visits. Many states already have telemedicine parity laws on the books where real-time telemedicine visits are required to be reimbursed at the exact same rate as in-person visits.

Going forward, since store-and-forward telemedicine visits take less time for physicians and generally offer the same results, we expect healthcare system to start favoring the faster store-and-forward visits whenever appropriate. In health systems where the hospital is also the health insurance provider, the physicians generally use the most cost-effective medical treatment technologies. Such mixed insurance and healthcare provider systems will be major drivers of best practices in telemedicine -- they are motivated by providing the patient with the best medical care in the most efficient way, and are less impacted by specific medical insurance regulations.

Attract New Patients and Grow the Market

Real-time telemedicine helps grow the overall market for patients. The reasons are the same as for store-and-forward telemedicine. By bringing medical treatment literally to the palm of the patient's hand, patients are more likely to seek treatment for issues they may have ignored or put off otherwise.

Real-time telemedicine offers a different engagement model than store-and-forward telemedicine, which will be more attractive to some patients. For optimal approach to attracting new patients, both real-time and store-and-forward options should be offered to patients. However, laws and insurance coverage in the medical provider's state may impact the most effective approach to rolling out telemedicine for new patients.

Challenges of Real-Time Telemedicine

The challenges, disadvantages, and risks of real-time telemedicine include:

- New Technology
- Potential distractions, including documentation requirements
- Scheduling issues
- No speed or timesaving advantages for medical providers
- Low video quality
- Being "on camera"
- Medical insurance coverage and malpractice insurance coverage
- Potential conflicts with existing patient interaction methods
- Staff training
- Integration with existing systems
- Cost

New Technology

Real-time telemedicine is considered a new technology for the same reasons as store-and-forward telemedicine. In addition, there are a couple features that add additional challenges to real-time telemedicine deployments.

An interactive telemedicine visit requires two sets of equipment to be set up and properly functional *at the same time*. Both parties must correctly set up the video camera, adjust the microphone, and ensure their Internet connection is working. Although this seems simple, in practice even frequent users occasionally fail.

We spent many years working with corporate managers who regularly hold audio and video meetings over the Internet. Time and time again, in a significant number of meetings, some technical issue would come up preventing one party from connecting. It could be a bad connection, the wrong meeting invitation, access issues, broken microphone, or a myriad of other causes. So, the meeting organizers would inevitably fiddle with the equipment for the first 5-10 minutes of the meeting, effectively wasting the time of the attendees. With some meeting organizers, things got so bad that attendees habitually began showing up at least 5 minutes late in the expectation of these issues. Several high level executives, in order to counteract this wasted time, required their administrative assistants to ensure all videoconference equipment was working ahead of time before they would even walk into a meeting.

Now, let's talk about those physicians and patients who may be much less tech savvy than the managers of high tech corporations. For patients, the real-time telemedicine visit will likely be the very first time they are using this particular telemedicine software. Even if they used the software before, it may have been several months ago and they can't be expected to remember all the tricks. Or maybe the software was upgraded since the last time they used it, so the user interface is different. Similarly, physicians will also need ramp up time – they will likely only see a few patients initially while getting the hang of the technology and fitting the new workflow into their existing practice. With both the patient and physician being relatively new users early in the telemedicine adoption process, the chances of something going wrong, whether user error or setup issue, will be fairly common. Meanwhile, during such hiccups, the physician will likely be in a middle of a busy day, while the patient may be anxious to get treatment. This only adds to the overall urgency and stress level when something doesn't work. When the real-time link can't be made, the cause of the issue may be as simple as a forgotten password. Yet the delay is twice as bad because it is time wasted for two parties.

Some real-time telemedicine vendors try to address the equipment setup issues by providing physicians with dedicated laptops to be used specifically for their telemedicine visits. The laptops are preconfigured and monitored by the telemedicine vendor's engineers to ensure a smooth experience for the physician. The dedicated laptops may also have a connection to the practice's EMR so that physician can readily input notes into the EMR during the virtual visit.

For the patient side, one way to ensure success is to ask the patient to make a test call to verify their audio and video setup. The test call can either be to a robot that simply takes a message and plays it back to the patient, or it could be to a live technician who manually verifies the connection. Depending on the precise software setup, the patient may be required to make the test call before being connected to the physician. In many implementations, patients must be the first ones to connect. They are then placed into a virtual waiting room, and the physician is notified that they have a telemedicine patient waiting.

Potential Distractions During Telemedicine Visit

Although real-time telemedicine is a very close proxy for an in-person visit, it is different in several important aspects. One difference is that both the patient and the physician are in front of their computer devices, with the inherent distractions that come with those devices. The distractions that we refer to include, but are not limited to:

- Email
- Text messages
- Social media sites such as Facebook and Twitter
- Web browsing

The patient, the physician, or both parties may not put their full and dedicated attention to the ongoing telemedicine visit.

The little pop up notification messages that come up for email, text messages, and others are called *toasts*. The reason they're called that is because in their first implementations, MSN Messenger and the Outlook email notification, the toast message came up from the bottom of the screen and popped out, much like a piece of bread pops out from a toaster. These and other types of interruptions easily draw attention away from the ongoing telemedicine visit. From our experience, many productivity gurus and coaches have endlessly criticized these types of interruptions. At **md Portal**, we have a saying about these notifications, directed at engineers and knowledge workers who need to focus on their current task: "If you don't disable toast messages, then you're toast!"

We have spoken to medical providers who regularly conduct phone and video telemedicine visits with their patients. The medical providers admit to occasionally checking email or browsing Facebook when conducting a real-time telemedicine visit. From our own experience in corporate culture, we've seen many, if not most, people with laptops try to multitask while attending a meeting. So such disengaging behavior during real-time telemedicine visits is not new, and not even unexpected. There are several possible reasons why physicians or patients may not be 100% engaged in a real-time telemedicine visit.

From the physician perspective, they often see the same conditions day in and day out. They know which questions to ask and what the typical patient responses are. Much of the time, physicians know what their patients will say. They have heard the most common responses, and they already know exactly what their next question will be to each of the common answer possibilities. Frequently, the physician generates a diagnosis and treatment plan within few minutes of interacting with the patient, long before the patient finishes telling their story. The only time physicians need to pay full attention is when a patient says something that either the medical provider has not heard before, or that may point to a rare condition. Thus, throughout most of the patient interview, many providers can effectively be on autopilot and do not need to be fully engaged.

The second reason for potential disengagement is the fact that the human brain is capable of taking in much more information than is presented in a typical real-time telemedicine visit, or any typical interaction for that matter. The average speaker speaks at a rate of 110 to 150 words per minute in a typical conversation. Meanwhile, the average reading speed is in the range of 200 to 300 words per minute. [26] Thus, the average human brain typically absorbs information twice as fast when reading as opposed to conversing. We speculate that during an interactive telemedicine visit, both the patient and physician may feel that they have spare brain bandwidth to multitask.

In contrast, the problem of slow speech has been solved for video and audio recordings in store-and-forward telemedicine applications. The top video and audio playback software allow users to adjust the speed of the playback, increasing the speed to 1.5 or 2 times the normal rate. The software automatically adjusts the sound pitch in the video, so that voices don't sound like cartoon characters. This playback speed technology is widespread – YouTube has been offering it for several years. When watching a YouTube video using the Chrome web browser, viewers can adjust the speed of the video from the settings menu.

This video speed up technology is widespread on university campuses, including medical schools. Many classes in medical school record their lectures so that students can watch or re-watch the lectures on their own time. Several medical school students we spoke with skip class on purpose for the sole purpose of saving time. Instead of going to class, they watch the recorded video lectures at a 1.5x or 2x sped up rate. In effect, they are selecting to receive education through store-and-forward telemedicine as opposed to a real-time interaction. In the similar vein, it may be faster for a physician to review a recorded video of their patient as opposed to have the interaction with the patient real-time.

Another opportunity for potential distraction during a real-time telemedicine visit is the requirement for documentation. Physicians must document the patient encounter for continuity of care and for insurance reimbursement. Since the physician is at their computer already, it makes sense for them to document the visit while the appointment is occurring. However, if the physician is not completely comfortable with their Electronic Medical Records (EMR) system, they may get distracted and tune out the patient. For example, when a patient mentions a unique type medical procedure they had, the physician may need figure out how to input that into the EMR. Additionally, assuming the medical provider is using a single monitor, both the patient telemedicine video and the EMR must share the same physical screen. So, if both the telemedicine and the EMR software applications cannot be reduced to half the screen size, or if physician chooses not to do so, then physician will not be seeing the patient while using their EMR because the EMR application will be on top of the video application. This may effectively reduce the experience for the physician to the level of a phone call.

Although it seems that all physicians should be familiar with their EMR, this is not the case in the real world. Many practices employ physical or virtual scribes to listen to the patient encounter and update the EMR, so that physician can focus their attention on the patient. Of course, if physician uses a scribe for the in-person visit, they may also use a scribe for the real-time telemedicine visit. The downside is the additional coordination required if the scribe is not in the same room as the physician. Holding a telemedicine visit between three parties adds another possibility for technical issues and additional scheduling requirements.

That said, for physicians who are proficient both with their EMR and with their telemedicine software, having both software applications on the same screen side-by-side may offer efficiency advantages. Because of that, some physicians may be able to complete and document interactive telemedicine visits faster than they can complete in-person visits.

Scheduling Issues

Unlike store-and-forward telemedicine, real-time telemedicine has a couple scheduling challenges that may impact patient satisfaction. For an interactive patient visit, both parties must be present at the same time. Some clinics using video telemedicine require that video visits be done during normal office hours. Physician may or may not be required to be physically present at the clinic for the visit (they may take the video visit from home). Because of these time restrictions, patients may not be able to complete a real-time telemedicine visit in the evening or weekend. Patients may need to interrupt their workday to do a video visit with their physician.

Another inherent issue that comes up when scheduling a real-time visit is that both parties may not actually be present during the appointed time of the visit. The physician could be running behind with their in-person patient visits, or the patient may have a workplace emergency. In the business world, two people with a scheduled virtual meeting sometimes play phone tag before their meeting starts. For example, the meeting time comes and one person is still held up in another meeting. They delay the start of their meeting. But then the second person has an impromptu call with another business associate, and the first person, after they free up, is left waiting as well.

Inevitably, one party or the other will be waiting for the visit to start. For some people and cultures, having the other party wait for them is a sign of power and respect. We speculate that some telemedicine patients may try their best to ensure that the physician is the one left waiting for them.

Typically, private practices optimize the clinic schedule for their providers to reduce or eliminate any dead time – if the provider is not seeing patients, then the clinic can't make money. When applied to video telemedicine visits, several strategies are employed to eliminate this scheduling friction for physicians:

- Provide the patient a window of time when their physician will call them
- Use medical staff or a receptionist to have the patient on the line before the visit – put the patient into a virtual waiting room
- If the patient is not present, charge them for the visit anyway

The first method gives patient a window of time, such as 2 hours, when the patient should wait by the phone or their device so that physician can contact them when they are ready. Occasionally, this window of time is very large, like a full day, which may be inconvenient for patients. This approach has a couple downsides. First, the patient may not be present when the physician calls. Second, patient may try to game the system by calling the practice to get a more precise time for the visit, and using up more of medical staff's time. Third, patient may take the call but require some additional time to find an isolated room where they can complete the visit with sufficient privacy.

The second approach, getting patient on the line, requires another person to be involved as well as keeps the patient waiting in a virtual exam room. Although one telemedicine advantage generally touted is that it requires less medical staff, in this case an additional staff person is needed to smooth out the visit for the physician. The staff person may either be an employee of the clinic or the telemedicine provider. On the patient side, if the patient is kept waiting on the line a significant amount of time, they may not see the point of doing a virtual video visit in the future, and choose to come in-person for their future appointments. After all, what's the point of waiting at the computer when you can wait in the physical waiting room?

The third approach of charging the patient regardless whether they show up, along with its cousin approaches of double booking and firing no-show patients, is a classic way to ensure that patients show up to their appointments. Patients generally do not appreciate such heavy-handed tactics to keep them in line.

Although we spent a lot of time above talking about potential scheduling issues and their impact on patient satisfaction, most of the above examples are corner cases. Generally speaking, they do not significantly detract from the patient advantages of convenience and eliminated travel.

No Speed or Timesaving Advantages for Medical Providers

When we speak to practicing physicians and practice managers, the biggest pushback to adopting real-time telemedicine visits by physicians is the lack of significant timesaving advantages. Real-time telemedicine shifts physician in-person visits to the Internet. Although real-time telemedicine offers flexibility, it does not readily allow physicians to see more patients in the same amount of time. Interactive telemedicine visits take approximately the same amount of time as in-person visits, they must be scheduled just like regular visits, and they are prone to the same types of cancellations and no-shows. While patients may receive huge savings from travel and wait times, many physicians, in contrast, do not view real-time telemedicine visits in the same favorable light.

What this means for established clinicians considering real-time telemedicine is that patient demand is by far the biggest consideration. Patients show their preference for real-time telemedicine by:

- Scheduling an interactive telemedicine visit over an in-person visit when given a choice (this may result in lower no-show rates for telemedicine visits)
- Switching to a practice that offers telemedicine

Store-and-forward telemedicine, in contrast, does provide distinct speed advantages for physicians. Even when store-and-forward video or audio is being employed, physicians in a hybrid practice are able to see more patients in the same amount of time. Hence, for an established practice that is at or near capacity, it makes sense to encourage new and existing patients to use store-and-forward virtual visits, and free up clinic time for additional patients, seeing them either in-person or through real-time telemedicine.

Low Video Quality

Video quality can be a challenge when using real-time video telemedicine. The beauty of real-time telemedicine is that patients and physicians can use their existing computers and mobile devices. However, that also means that some users will use high quality video cameras while other users will use older lower quality cameras.

Besides the camera, another important factor impacting video quality is the Internet connection. Patients and physicians using mobile devices must rely on wireless Wi-Fi or the cellular data connection from their mobile provider. These connections typically have higher latencies and lower bandwidth than landline connections, and they may not be able to support a high quality video stream. Even if one party uses a high quality fiber connection, the overall video quality will be largely dictated by the slower connection -- the weak link in the chain. If the patient uses a mobile device with a bad connection, they may see a low quality jerky video of their physician. This is because the patient's download speed will be slow. And the doctor on the other end will see a low quality image of the patient because the patient's upload speed will also be slow.

Although extremely poor and jerky video connection is intolerable for just abound anyone, a smooth low-resolution video may not be an issue for some specialties and use cases. For example, holding a real-time video visit for the primary purpose of educating the patient should work just fine with a lower resolution. In contrast, using real-time video with a dermatologist can be a challenge – patient trying to show their physician a rash on their arm may not be able to provide a good enough picture or angle for a medical diagnosis.

Clinics can take several measures to mitigate the possibility of poor video during visits. First, physicians must always use a good connection for their video visits, either in the clinic or at their home. Next, clinics should ask patients to use a good video connection. As mentioned earlier, patients should do a test call before the visit to check both their overall setup and video quality. Third, video visits requiring high quality images, such as dermatology, should be supplemented with store-and-forward technologies.

Telemedicine Combination of Both Store-and-Forward and Real-Time

Let's take a moment to discuss compound telemedicine approaches, specifically using both real-time and store-and-forward telemedicine in a single visit. Either before or after the real-time telemedicine interaction, the patient can asynchronously provide additional information to their physician. This information may include not only common items such as allergies and medical history, but also questionnaires specific to the condition and supplemental image upload. Even if video quality is excellent, a patient's problem area may physically be difficult to show with a video camera, in which case a photo is needed. For example, the problem area may be on the patient's leg, and the camera they're using may be attached to a stationary desktop computer. Just imagine the headlines if the patient was always required to show their hard to reach areas for the video camera: "Patient Injures Themselves While Trying to Contort for a Telemedicine Visit." For a physician, having all of the clinical data up front before the real-time portion of the appointment is preferable, since then the diagnosis can be made right away and next steps communicated to the patient. However, in rare cases additional information may be needed after the visit (more pictures, etc.) for a specific diagnosis.

Offering a compound store-and-forward and real-time virtual visit gains some of the benefits from both types of telemedicine. The store-and-forward component provides speed advantages for the physician, while the real-time portion of the visit provides immediate feedback and potential insurance advantages. The interactive part of the compound visit should be much shorter than if the entire visit was real-time. The entire patient history and any pictures should already be available before the real-time interaction starts. The medical interview should be short to non-existent.

In many situations, a compound model is more preferable than real-time or store-and-forward solution stand-alone. State laws, medical insurance, and malpractice insurance requirements may exclude store-and-forward telemedicine as an option for some types of care models, such as new patient initial visits. Thus, the real-time component may be required to meet insurance and regulation requirements, even if the medical provider does not deem the real-time portion medically necessary. In such cases, the physician may simply provide their findings, education, and next steps during the video portion, without asking for additional information from the patient.

The downside of the compound approach is the additional complexity it adds for both the clinic and the patient. Patients may need additional support while going through the virtual visit flow, and physicians must be proficient in both types of telemedicine approaches.

Being "on camera"

Now, let's discuss being "on camera", a challenge unique to real-time telemedicine. We're referring here to the video camera on physician's mobile device or computer. In medical schools, traditional training covers face-to-face interaction with patients. That said, a few people may argue this training isn't done very well due to the poor bedside manners of some physicians. In either case, it is safe assume that most established clinicians have an inordinate amount of experience interacting with patients in the cozy comfort of the exam room.

Completing a real-time telemedicine visit, on the other hand, is akin to being on a reality television show. Effectively, this means the physician is a reality TV actor. Taking the situation to the extreme, the patient, on the other end, could theoretically be recording the interaction for the expressed purpose of later uploading it to YouTube. While in the exam room with an in-person patient, the physician could make a minor slip up and no one would be the wiser. For example, forgetting a minor side effect of a medication. But if the physician slips up during a real-time telemedicine visit, their real-life exploits might not only reach a national audience, but also increase their legal liability. And what if a potential patient peruses the practice's Yelp reviews and encounters an out-of-context picture or video from a real-time telemedicine visit? If that hasn't happened yet, then it's just a matter of time.

Let's not beat around the bush – having a recordable video of the physician is great for patients, at least in the long term. However, it adds additional liability for the physician and their practice. By taking the medical consultation out of the brick-and-mortar exam room, patients are given more power. Power, that, at least in some cases, patients may not be able to properly handle.

People are generally nicer when they communicate in person. However, away from that direct face-to-face contact, either on the phone or in online chat rooms, many people tend to make much more aggressive remarks and inflammatory statements. In one example on Facebook, an ER physician made a comment about his experience in response to a newspaper article on the dangers of pit bulls. Tons of people piled on with criticism, personally attacking and trying to discredit the doctor. The doctor unfriended the original poster of the article and broke all contact with her. [27]

But aren't patients generally nice when they see their doctor? When patients come to the doctor's office, they come to a place surrounded by uniformed personnel with a special waiting area separating them from the clinic staff. Before seeing a doctor, they may be asked to undress and put on a hospital gown. Many patients are intimidated and act docile in such an environment. In fact, it is well known that some patients feel anxiety and their blood pressure readings are higher when they are in the doctor's office. It is called white coat syndrome. Of course, that's not true of all patients. Many patients visiting the doctor may have mental health issues and may not behave like everyone else. About 20% of the visits to a primary care provider are mental health-related, not counting the cases where a mental health issue was not disclosed or discovered. [28] Other patients may behave differently due to other factors, such as chronic pain or the frustration of the long wait to see their doctor.

Sufficient behavioral psychology studies comparing face-to-face and video interaction have not been done. Nevertheless, with the change of environment and other factors, we believe it is safe to assume that, at least for some patients, the physician-patient conversation over real-time telemedicine will be significantly different than the face-to-face counterpart. Why do people behave differently online than face-to-face? There are several theories. First, since the parties are not in physical contact with each other, there is no chance of physical harm, which has an emboldening effect on some individuals. Second, since people are interacting through machines and not directly with touchable human beings, the interaction may not feel "real" for some people, meaning that, to a certain degree, their actions may not feel to have consequences. Third, in many online situations people are anonymous for the expressed or implied purpose of communicating thoughts that they otherwise wouldn't if their identity was known.

Now, is anonymity really a problem for telemedicine, where physicians should know the identity of their patient? Not exactly. But a related problem may be. Sometimes patients visit a doctor with a complaint that they actually don't have. They're often simply trying to get medication for themselves or for their friend. Anecdotally speaking, this is what many people do in California to get a prescription for marijuana – pretend they have certain symptoms. With telemedicine making it easier to connect patients and medical providers, the incidence of fraudulent complaints will rise. Perhaps we should call these fake complaints what they are – prank telemedicine calls.

Ok, enough talk about the patients misbehaving. What about the physicians -- aren't physicians going to act differently online than they do in real life? Yes. And that's part of the reasons why we're bringing up being "on camera" – physicians may need training and practice to develop a great "stage presence". Physicians are professionals living in the 21st century, where practically anything people do could be recorded. It is pointless to "hide behind a rock" and pretend the reality of social and technological advancements is somehow outside the realm of medical practice. We speculate that some patients may come to their doctor's office wearing Google Glass for the expressed purpose of streaming their visit. So, physicians may increasingly be "on camera" even during face-to-face visits.

Being "on camera" means the patient can only see the physician through their screen – they can't see what the physician is doing off screen or outside the frame. This means basic human interactions, from introductions to the actual exam, if any, are fundamentally different. Communication must be directed at the camera, eye contact should be maintained with the camera and not with the computer screen, and any hand gestures must also be in front of the camera. When starting out with telemedicine, we recommend physicians to record their virtual visits. This way, they can get price feedback about how their telemedicine patients see them. Yes, it may be extremely uncomfortable to see and hear yourself on-screen. However, that may be the best way to improve "stage presence" and offer the best care for your patients.

Medical Insurance Coverage and Malpractice Insurance Coverage

Let's move on to the next challenge for real-time telemedicine, which is medical insurance coverage for patients and malpractice insurance coverage for physicians. These challenges are similar for all types of telemedicine, including store-and-forward and remote monitoring. States have been regularly issuing new laws in this area, which have been generally favorable to telemedicine, and to real-time telemedicine in particular. In the next several years, we expect laws across all 50 states to be fairly consistent as far as acceptance and availability of real-time and other categories of telemedicine.

Conflict with Existing Patient Interaction Methods

The next challenge with adopting real-time telemedicine is the conflict with existing methods. We covered this topic when discussing store-and-forward telemedicine. In addition to reconciling on-call and patient portal interactions with patients, some clinics may provide both real-time and store-and-forward telemedicine options for their patients. Depending on reimbursement policies and other factors, real-time telemedicine may be favorable for some care models while store-and-forward favorable for others. Reputable telemedicine vendors should provide clinics with suggestions and recommendations regarding reconciling their virtual interactions with patients based on the clinic's specialty, state of location, and the supported care models.

Staff Training, Integration with Existing Systems, and Cost

Staff training, integration with existing systems, and cost are additional challenges that are common for both store-and-forward and real-time telemedicine. These challenges have already been covered in detail in the chapter on store-and-forward telemedicine. For training, medical staff and physicians must be trained on the new real-time system, including the setup of the videoconferencing portions.

Integration with existing systems may or may not be needed depending on the available features of the real-time telemedicine system. For example, if the real-time telemedicine system only consists of Skype-like functionality and does not hold any patient medical information, then no integration is needed. The clinic can schedule patients in their existing scheduling system, request patients to use their existing billing system, and physician can make visit notes directly in the EMR. For patient visit reminders, the clinic staff can call the patient or use another third-party service, similar to what is done for in-person visits. One caveat is that during this reminder call, clinic staff may ensure the patient's software is set up and provide the patient with any additional instructions.

Conversely, if the real-time telemedicine system does include patient medical information, scheduling, e-prescribing, and other features, then it should be electronically or manually integrated with existing systems to keep all clinic's information consistent. Scheduling in particular must be integrated with the clinic's existing in-person scheduling system. Clinics should not unintentionally double book virtual real-time visits with in-person visits.

Remote Monitoring

In this chapter we cover the type of telemedicine categorized as remote monitoring. The primary feature of remote patient monitoring is the use of sensors for measuring patient body's functions such as heart rate, blood pressure, and temperature while the patient is away from the healthcare facility. Typical deployment locations for remote monitoring technologies are a patient's home or a community-living center such as a nursing home.

The sensor data is gathered regularly, either automatically or through manual steps. Fully automated sensors use intelligent software and hardware to upload their data to a central system that can be accessed by a physician, with little to no additional interaction by the patient. For example, certain types of pacemakers send their data to another local device, often called a *sensor hub*, which then streams the data over the Internet, uploading it to remote monitoring application servers. Other sensors require a manual step to get the sensor measurements into the system, such as synchronization with a computer by plugging in the device or manual data entry for completely stand-alone devices.

Remote monitoring technologies are often used together with store-and-forward or real-time telemedicine. Many patients using remote monitoring have chronic conditions requiring regular and frequent follow-ups with their physician. As covered in the previous chapters, completing the follow-up via store-and-forward or real-time telemedicine is a convenience for patients. Also, for patients who have been advised not to travel, doing a virtual visit may be the best possible option.

Over the last several years, we've seen an explosion of new biosensing wearables onto the market. [10] Wearable sensors are available for many body functions, including:

- Movement
- Heart rate
- Sleep
- Temperature
- Respiration
- Skin conductance
- Brain activity
- Hydration
- Posture
- Glucose
- Oxygen level
- Heart rate variability
- Muscle activity
- Blood pressure

Besides wearable sensors, stationary devices can also be used to perform different body measurements, such as scales for weight and traditional blood pressure cuffs for blood pressure. Other types of sensors do not measure the body directly but instead measure a patient's location. In a community-living facility, physicians and staff can monitor patient's indoor location by using technologies such as RFID or Bluetooth iBeacon. Such local location technologies can be useful to assess patient activity as well as to find the patient quickly in case of emergency.

Monitoring of movement and activity is perhaps the most common type of remote monitoring today. Accelerometer, the sensor type used for activity tracking, is present in practically all modern mobile phone devices. This sensor can be used to monitor movement patterns and even sudden falls for mobility-challenged patients. We witnessed a demonstration of a beta phone app for detecting falls and stumbles.

Centers for Medicare & Medicaid Services (CMS) and major insurance providers are now covering remote patient monitoring. Like other forms of telemedicine, the coverage has been expanding in recent years. The current procedural terminology (CPT) code 99091 covers collecting and reviewing patient data. When combining chronic care management and remote patient monitoring, the monthly fee to providers is approximately $100. [29]

Behavioral Monitoring

Another type of monitoring that has seen recent growth is behavioral monitoring. For patients with mental illness and those at risk for depression, behavioral monitoring can catch early signs of mental issues and allow intervention as soon as possible. Since many people carry a mobile device with them, some monitoring solutions are using software running on the patient's mobile device to automatically track patient behavior, including integrating with any other sensors that are present on the device. Mobile devices are continuously becoming more powerful by integrating new sensors such as pedometers and new functionalities such as indoor location tracking. Out of the box, most modern mobile phone devices can be used to track the following behavioral activities:

- Location
- Phone calls and text messages sent/received, including identity of the other party and total conversation time
- Time spent using specific applications and browsing web sites
- Approximate sleep time, based on accelerometer activity and time of day

In addition, behavior-tracking apps can automatically prompt patients on a regular basis to answer a questionnaire about their current state or manually log their mood. The apps can also provide immediate feedback such as reminding patients to take a walk or to speak to someone in their support group if they haven't done so recently.

Monitoring in Emergency Medicine

In addition to tracking patients at home, another use case for remote monitoring is emergency medicine. Let's take an example of a paramedic assisted by telemedicine technology. When arriving at the scene, the paramedic may use the following devices:

- Cardiometer
- Defibrillator
- Oximeter
- ECG Monitor

All of these devices may be connected to a remote monitoring system, so that physicians at the hospital can monitor the patient at the scene, or monitor the patient while they are being transported to the hospital. In addition, the paramedic may wear a video camera and send the real-time telemedicine feed of what they are seeing to the hospital.

Personal Fitness Monitoring

With the explosion of new sensors on the market, the biggest growth area for remote monitoring has been personal fitness and general health assessments. These areas generally fall outside of the prevue of traditional medicine, as they involve already healthy individuals maintaining or improving their fitness.

The most popular personal fitness sensor is a pedometer, which tracks the number of steps a person takes. Fitbit, the maker of a prominent movement and activity monitor, has seen tremendous demand and filed for an IPO (Initial Public Offering) in May of 2015. [11] The company began trading on NASDAQ in June of 2015. Many modern mobile devices are now jumping into the fitness trend and including built in pedometer functionality in their offerings. The generally acceptable recommendation is that a person should take at least 10,000 steps per day for a healthy lifestyle. Other popular fitness sensors measure heart rate and sleep. Sleep sensors measure the person's movement during sleep to determine the quality and duration of sleep. Sleep monitors can be used to help identify what external factors help get a good night's sleep or cause a sleepless night.

Although personal fitness may not necessarily be medically significant for a single individual, it may be significant for population health. With the rising costs of healthcare, companies and organizations are looking for ways to improve the health of their employees. They see fitness tracking as a proxy for improving health and happiness of their employees, increasing productivity, decreasing sick time, and reducing overall medical expenses. Organizations are encouraging their members to use wearable fitness sensors and other monitoring technology by:

- Giving insurance discounts and prizes to members achieving certain fitness monitor usage goals
- Holding competitions between departments for total steps walked
- Offering free consultations with a health coach who monitors the member's activity data
- Giving public recognition to members actively tracking their fitness

Thus, remote patient monitoring is not just for people with medical conditions. It is actively being used for healthy, and even extremely fit individuals.

Benefits of Remote Monitoring

In the next sections, we discuss the advantages and challenges of deploying and using remote monitoring technologies. A few of the advantages and challenges are the same as for store-and-forward and/or real-time telemedicine. For these items, since they were discussed in detail in the previous chapters, we will only call out any factors unique to remote patient monitoring.

The advantages and benefits of remote patient monitoring include:

- Convenience
- Reduced hospital stay, lower re-admission rates, fewer ER visits
- Increased patient compliance
- Early alerts of patient's change of condition, faster response, and accurate triage
- Detailed and frequent history of patient's vital signs and other body measurements
- Peace of mind for patient's family members
- Reduced liability due to completely digital audit trail
- Easier physician education and consults

Convenience

Patient and physician convenience is the hallmark benefit of telemedicine. For remote patient monitoring, the convenience for patients is that they can take their vital signs and other body function measurements from the comfort of their home, without traveling to a healthcare facility. From a medical provider perspective, all necessary patient measurements are accessible on a secure Internet site. These measurements are either available in real-time or on a regular basis, depending on the technologies used. Since the data is readily available, the physician does not need to spend as much time questioning the patient or taking additional in-office measurements in order to assess the patient's progress. In addition, for patients who cannot travel, a medical professional does not need to visit the patient at their place of residence to take these measurements.

Reduced Hospital Stay and Lower Re-Admission Rates

The next benefits of remote patient monitoring are reduced hospital stays and lower re-admission rates. Sometimes patients must stay in the hospital so that the hospital staff can closely monitor their condition. With remote monitoring technologies, if patient's vitals and other body function measurements can be monitored remotely, the patient may be discharged much earlier. In many cases, this improves the quality of life for the patient by getting them out of the hospital. For the hospital, it frees up a bed for potentially more serious cases.

With remote patient monitoring, the re-admission rates may be lower because potential issues can be caught earlier before the problem is severe enough to require re-admission. For example, if the patient's physiological inputs are not trending in the right direction, the physician can adjust patient medication, potentially preventing a re-admission.

Increased Patient Compliance

In many cases, the remote monitoring measurements may be trending in the wrong direction because the patient is not adhering to their medication regimen. Patients who don't adhere to their medication are 17% more likely to visit the emergency room and 10% more likely to be readmitted. [30] Identifying such non-compliant patients as early as possible is extremely helpful, since it gives medical professionals time to target interventions, such as:

- Additional patient education and health coaching

- Alerts and reminders to take medication
- Ensure sufficient supply of medication is available; possibly using a mail-order pharmacy so the patient does not need to travel for refills
- Economic incentives for compliant patients such as lottery drawings
- Adjusting medication regimens so that they're easier to follow, such as synchronizing the time for taking multiple medications

Many hospitals and health systems are financially incentivized to reduce re-admission rates. Increasing patient compliance using remote patient monitoring is a cost-effective way to help achieve these goals.

Early Alerts

As mentioned above, remote patient monitoring lets physician see changes in patient's body function measurements fairly frequently. With some telemedicine systems, automatic alerts can be set up so the physician receives a text message, phone call, or email if certain changes in the patient's body measurements are detected. When remote monitoring sensors provide a real-time data stream, the alerts can be real-time as well.

For example, medically accurate sensors that measure ECG, heart rate, and other cardiovascular functions will soon be readily available. A patient with increased risk for a heart attack may be instructed to use their at-home ECG sensor to take a measurement when they experience chest pains. Then, a medical provider will get an alert, log into the remote monitoring system, and triage this heart event to detect whether it is something that requires immediate medical intervention and hospitalization, or whether it is something that can wait until the next regular physician visit.

Overall, all of today's wearable devices and sensors are becoming more and more accurate, approaching the quality of in-office equipment. In addition, as more types of sensors are appearing on the market, more body functions can be measured. The above-mentioned market forces are creating an unprecedented ability to see what's happening with the patient's body at or near real-time. As the overall trends continue, these devices will become even more accurate, more convenient, less invasive, and longer lasting. This means additional types of patients and conditions will be eligible for remote monitoring. And, once the volumes are high enough, we speculate that dedicated patient monitoring centers will spring up, with medical providers working in shifts and being specially trained for remote monitoring, much like dedicated off-site centers exist today for teleradiology.

Detailed Measurement History Available for Analysis

Remote patient monitoring systems digitally store patient measurements for several years, depending on the telemedicine vendor's policies and state requirements. Having a detailed historical view of patient body's functions allows physicians access to analytics, and allows them to run correlations to determine:

- What events impact the patient's health for better or worse
- What a patient's best day looks like
- What are he long term impacts of specific medical regiments or procedures
- How does patient compare to their peers
- Which medical interventions consistently achieve the best outcomes

Having detailed data from their own patient population allows physicians to see trends across different conditions, regiments, and age groups. This allows physicians to use evidence-based medicine from their own patients to adjust their approach.

Peace of Mind for Patient's Family

When a patient is hospitalized or has a chronic condition, that patient's family members are concerned and often want as much information as possible. When patient remote monitoring is used, family members can be given access to the telemedicine application to see the patient's data feed and any alerts. This gives them piece of mind for knowing as much as possible about their loved one, as well as gives them the opportunity to be closely involved with the care. If the family members are willing, they can even be given additional responsibilities, such as:

- Watching for specific danger signs
- Manually updating the telemedicine application for certain types of measurements and information
- Helping with patient compliance

These activities can be done even if the family members are not co-located with the patient. For example, children of elderly patients often live in another city due to work or other requirements. Thus, remote patient monitoring allows not only physicians, but also patient's family to be involved in the treatment.

Digital Audit Trail

The last but not least advantages of remote patient monitoring are reduced liability due to digitally stored information and easier physician education and consults. These are the same advantages we already discussed for store-and-forward telemedicine. In both store-and-forward and remote monitoring telemedicine applications, all patient information is generally stored in perpetuity, and the entire patient encounter (or a series of encounters) can effectively be *replayed*.

For some types of remote monitoring data streams, especially ones that generate a lot of data, the software vendor may choose to compress the older measurements by only keeping several summary indicators. The increase in the number of sensors on the market and the improvement in accuracy of existing sensors guarantee that more and more remote patient monitoring data will be generated in the future. At the same time, the high tech industry is ramping up for the expected growth of the Internet of Things (IoT). The IoT supporters expect many smaller devices and sensors, such as light bulbs and thermometers, to be connected to the Internet and streaming data between each other and to the cloud.

The IoT movement and the expectant increase in the amount of generally-available sensor data has spurred on improvements in computing infrastructure, including dedicated databases for time-series data, such as InfluxDB. [31] Some software vendors offer solutions for storing IoT sensor data without loss – keeping all of the data forever. This Internet "cat and mouse game" of more data and better ways to store and organize this data has been happening for years and, in our opinion, will continue into the foreseeable future.

Challenges of Remote Monitoring

Now, let's switch to the more critical side. The disadvantages and challenges of remote patient monitoring include:

- Patient training and patient cost
- Dizzying array of devices to choose from
- Patient inconvenience and lower quality of life (loss of independence and loss of privacy)
- Sensor device accuracy and reliability
- Getting consistent data from different sensors
- Too much data
- Staff training
- Integration with existing systems
- Health provider cost

Patient Training and Patient Cost

The first challenge of remote patient monitoring is patient training. In a typical remote monitoring deployment, physician may want to track several measurements. Let's take a simple demonstration of heart rate and weight. A common example of a heart rate sensor is a device worn on the wrist that streams data to the patient's mobile device or computer, which then transfers the measurements to the cloud. Weight, meanwhile, can be tracked manually by using a common scale and updating a web form. Also, weight can also be tracked semi-automatically – electronic weight scales are now available that send their measurements to another device or directly to the cloud. The reason they track weight "semi-automatically" is because today the patient actually has to step on the scale to get their weight. In our opinion, future smart homes will be able to measure occupant's weight in real-time using smart pressure-sensing floors.

Before enabling all the monitoring data streams, the patient must be acquainted with the devices they will use. This includes instructions for:

- Wearing the actual device
- Taking measurements
- Uploading the data to the telemedicine system

- Maintaining the device and charging its battery
- Additional special instructions (for example, carrying the mobile phone with them if the phone is part of the overall patient monitoring solution)

Training takes time. Some devices are easier to use than others. In addition, many patients, especially the elderly patients most in need of remote monitoring, may have difficulty grasping all the process steps to transfer data, or may be physically incapable of operating small sensors without additional help. Thus, even when patient is equipped with all the proper sensors and sent home, the remote monitoring may fail due to user error or insufficient training.

In addition, medical insurance may not cover the actual monitoring devices, so the patient may need to pay out of pocket. The physician office may have the devices available for purchase or the office staff could direct the patient to a nearby retail location. Some patients may choose to order the devices online due to reduced costs, resulting in a delay before starting the monitoring. Training at the healthcare facility could be a challenge when the actual devices the patient will use aren't on-hand.

Many Devices on the Market

The next issue, and something we've alluded to already, is that there is a dizzying array of devices to choose from, and new offerings from new vendors are constantly being release. Although this is a benefit because it presents additional care opportunities, this is also a challenge when selecting the specific devices for a specific patient. The clinic or hospital may have a set of devices that they either recommend or that patients are required to choose from. However, many electronic devices don't stay on the market long. And even with preferred devices, the physicians must keep up with the constant updates and new models coming out from the vendors. In addition, since many patients will be paying out of pocket for their own measurement devices, they may want to use another device. Or, as the prevalence of devices increases, patients may even want to use an older device that they already have. Maybe they got it free from a friend of theirs as a birthday present. If the practice plans to use remote monitoring for a significant number of patients, we recommend assigning a dedicated staff member who can help patients with the device onboarding process.

Patient Inconvenience and Lower Quality of Life

The next challenge with remote monitoring is quality of life. Yes, we know -- this is both a benefit and a challenge. The benefit is that remote monitoring potentially allows the patient early discharge from the hospital. The challenge is that many wearable devices and sensors are inconvenient, and the patient loses a level of independence by being constantly watched by "Big Brother". Many sensors must be worn on the wrist, ankle, or torso throughout the day and night. The sensors may interfere with patient's other clothing, get in the way while sleeping, and may need to be continuously taken off and put back on for showering and other activities. Although, as with most things in life, the patient will eventually get accustomed to their remote monitored lifestyle, expect hic-ups along the way. If the devices initially frustrate patients, some of them may flat out refuse to use remote monitoring.

As Atul Gawande explains in *Being Mortal*, nursing homes and other elderly care providers often market their services to the children of the patient and not to the patient themselves, since these facilities know that it is the children of the patient who are often driving the decision. [32] In a similar fashion, we expect that much of the demand for patient monitoring may be driven by patient's family and not necessarily by the actual patient or even by the their physician. Loss of independence may trigger depression and other illnesses in many people. And accepting remote monitoring may indicate to many patients that they can't take care of themselves. Thus, it is important to have the patient's full cooperation when instituting remote patient monitoring. In some cases, even if technology is otherwise available, the amount of monitoring may need to be reduced in order to allow the patient as much independence and self-sufficiency as possible.

Monitoring Device Accuracy and Reliability

The next challenge with remote patient monitoring is device accuracy and reliability. Although we mentioned an explosion of device sensors in the market, most such devices are targeted directly at consumers without being classified as medical devices.

In the United States, a medical device is defined as a device intended for diagnosis, treatment, or prevention of a medical condition. Devices that work through chemical action inside or on the human body are characterized as drugs and fall under different laws and classifications. Medical devices must be recognized and approved by the Food and Drug Administration (FDA). There are three classes of medical devices – Class I, Class II, and Class III. Class I are convenience devices not substantially important to human health, while Class III are devices that support or sustain human life. Some types of devices, like those designed to detect a heart attack, may need to be classified as Class III. The FDA approval process may be expensive and lengthy, and not all device manufacturers may be willing to go through it. The FDA approval for Withing's Smart Body Scale took over two years. [33] In addition, if the new device is not substantially equivalent to a previously FDA-approved device, then clinical trials may be required, just like for new drug approvals. The clinical trial expense may be prohibitive for some companies and types of devices – for example, the market (patients, physicians, insurance companies) may not be willing to pay a high enough price for the device to justify clinical trials.

The good news is that medical providers are allowed to prescribe non-medical devices for their patients. For example, a physician may prescribe a standing desk to a patient suffering from backaches. The key point here is that if the FDA did not approve this standing desk as a medical device, the standing desk manufacturer cannot claim it helps with back pain or any other medical condition. However, if the manufacturer decides to market the desk as a back pain reliever, they must get FDA approval before doing so. So, in essence, many devices on the market can be used to treat medical conditions even though they cannot explicitly state so due to FDA regulations. So, you may ask, why does a physician even bother by paying attention to the medical device regulations? By prescribing a non-medical non-FDA approved device, the physician takes on additional liability. This means if the patient injures themselves when using the non-medical device prescribed by the physician, they may have a stronger court case against their provider. Their case may be even stronger if an FDA-approved alternative device was available. Almost all physicians carry medical liability insurance, and, in our experience, any reputable medical liability insurance would cover such medical negligence cases. Medical liability insurances typically only exclude coverage for conduct that is illegal, such as altering records or theft.

There is a "chicken and the egg" dilemma here. To be attractive, patient monitoring must be cheap. However, the expenses associated with FDA approval process may cause device prices to be out of reach for many patients. What we currently see in the industry is that although any physician can look at data generated from non-FDA approved devices, many will not make any medical decisions based on that data and instead will use their own established methods to effectively duplicate and verify the results. Due to liability concerns, some physicians we encountered do not trust measurements taken by other health professionals -- it is common practice for physicians to request that some of patient tests and measurements be redone by a clinic's approved lab. Even with medical liability insurance coverage, being sued is still a hassle, and many medical providers take all the precautions they can.

Using non-FDA approved remote monitoring devices for medically significant tasks is completely out of the question for many physicians. For example, using a non-FDA approved electrocardiogram (ECG) app to determine if patient must receive immediate medical attention. In such cases, we expect that many physicians will not trust the software and either use traditional methods or always direct the patient to the emergency room.

One piece of good news is that, in 2014, FDA proposed deregulation for certain types of measurement devices such as thermometers, smart body scales, stethoscopes, ophthalmic cameras, and others. [34] Although this recommendation must go through the normal ratification process, this signals a huge boost to the remote monitoring industry. Physicians and telemedicine vendors will soon have many more device options to choose from, and to be able to use them for medically significant decisions. Device vendors will be able to sell new devices in these categories for direct integration into patient monitoring platforms without waiting for lengthy approvals.

If the patient is already tracking their own health with remote monitoring devices, looking at the data can be a good way to get a general sense of the patient's health. For many people we spoke with, the usage of the device in the first place without a specific medical recommendation may indicate that the patient is strongly motivated to be healthy.

Many physicians and general public view the data generated by FDA-approved devices to be more accurate and reliable than data generated by similar non-approved sensors. This is not necessarily true. The measurement tolerances are listed in the device specifications, and many non-FDA approved devices may in fact be more accurate than the FDA-approved versions.

Although the overall news and trends are favorable for wide acceptance of remote monitoring devices, physicians and telemedicine providers must keep in mind that there will always be variability between devices, measurement noise, and environmental factors that affect each measurement. Thus, physicians must always be more cautious when reviewing the data from remote monitoring devices, and ensure ahead of time that the accuracy is sufficient for diagnostic purposes. Additionally, measurement accuracy and reliability may be impacted not only by the sensor itself, but also by the related infrastructure. Once the sensor measurement is taken, the data often needs to flow through multiple data hubs before reaching a central database. If any of those links are down, which can easily happen when, for example, patient loses Internet connection, only partial or inaccurate data may be uploaded, and the "whole picture" may not be readily visible to the physician.

Getting Consistent Data from Different Sensors

The next challenge to discuss is integrating the data from multiple sensors and displaying it in one place using a consistent format. Many devices may generate the same measurement, like body temperature, but the data stream may be formatted differently. We'll use the measurement of temperature in our examples to demonstrate the point. Listed below are a few ways data streams measuring essentially the same thing may be different:

- Rate of measurement (how many times per hour?)
- Number of significant digits
- Location of measurement
- Type of measurement technology
- Post processing filters

For rate of measurement, one device may take measurements once a minute, another device may take measurements once every 10 minutes, and yet a third device may take measurements whenever the user presses its "take a measurement" button. A medical provider may have patients using all three types of these devices. Yet when they take a look at the remote patient monitoring dashboard, they expect to see the data in a consistent format.

The number of significant digits is the accuracy of the sensor – one temperature sensor may state 98.6°F while another sensor may state 98.58°F.

The location of measurement is where the measurement is physically being taken – wrist, hip, chest, ear, rectum, head, or some other body part. Different parts of the body may be at different temperatures depending on the environment, clothing, and other factors. For example, when people are in a chilly environment, their hands and feet may be a lower temperature than the rest of their body.

The measurement technology is the physical type of sensor being used to take the measurement. Manufacturers may use different sensor types due to their cost, size, ruggedness, convenience, and other factors. Temperature can be measured with contact or non-contact sensors. Contact temperature sensors include:

- Thermocouples

- Resistance Temperature Detectors (RTDs)
- Thermistors

Non-contact temperature measurements, on the other hand, can be done with infrared sensors.

Many measurement devices perform processing or filtering of the data stream before actually sending the data to the end user. This additional step is often needed to improve accuracy or reduce environmental noise. A simple example of post processing is the average – the device may take 10 measurements in a single minute, average them, and send back a single number with an additional significant digit. What this means in this example is that the data is actually slightly delayed due to the time needed to take multiple measurements. Other post processing tricks may include dropping measurements flagged as noisy and adjusting the measurement based on environmental conditions known to impact the sensors, such as humidity or pressure.

When putting together a system for efficiently reviewing patient remote monitoring data, telemedicine vendors and medical providers should consider the above-mentioned variations when collecting the same measurement type. The technical term for converting data of different formats into the same format is called **normalization**. Several companies are offering normalization services for sensor data, such as Human API and Validic.

Too Much Data

In addition to data normalization, another challenge is the sheer volume of data and the ability to sift through it all. One issue is simply showing multiple measurement types on a single dashboard -- even after the data is normalized, it must be displayed in a convenient and physician-friendly format. Furthermore, some measurement types may be more medically relevant than others. Unfortunately, from our experience, many of today's biosensor data aggregation systems are still primarily focused on keeping up with supporting all the current and upcoming sensors on the market, and less with organizing, searching, and extracting medically relevant insights from the data.

Another issue caused by the sheer volume of data is the increased number of false positives. If a physician is looking for a specific data anomaly, such as a dip in patient breathing rate, such anomalies may happen multiple times throughout the day. Many are likely caused by environment or special situations, such as excitement from watching a movie, and do not necessarily signal a change in the patient's medical condition. In the worst case, the medical provider or caregiver may set up an alert for these anomalies, then receive way too many alerts, and, as a result, begin to disregard them. Ignoring alerts may then miss a legitimate medical issue. Instead, notification alerts must be set up with the up-front consideration regarding the number of false positives likely to be triggered. The most sophisticated data aggregation remote monitoring systems are able to take multiple factors into account before triggering a notification, such as time of day, length of anomaly, and other related measurements.

Staff Training, Integration, and Health Provider Cost

The last challenges with remote patient monitoring are the same types of challenges that we already discussed in the chapters on store-and-forward and real-time telemedicine – staff training, integration with existing systems, and cost.

When integrating with existing systems, remote monitoring is often used alongside real-time and store-and-forward telemedicine approaches. In addition to being remotely monitored, the patient may also have real-time video check-ins with their medical staff. Thus, patient monitoring and data aggregation may not only need to be integrated with existing clinic systems, but also with another telemedicine system. Many existing telemedicine vendors are viewing patient monitoring and general health monitoring as a natural expansion of their service offerings. Thus, expect future telemedicine products to include patient monitoring functionality fully integrated with their existing systems.

Selecting a Telemedicine Technology Vendor

In the early-to-mid 2000s, most medical offices ran on paper medical records. [35] [36] The move from paper records to electronic medical records (EMRs) was long and arduous. In many ways, it may be a preview for the upcoming mass move from in-person patient visits to a hybrid mix of telemedicine and in-person visits. In other ways, the move to hybrid practices will be much smoother. After the transition to electronic records, many office managers have learned their lessons and will not make the same mistakes. The key suggestions coming out of the EMR move, which also apply to telemedicine adoption, include:

- Receiving buy-in and feedback from medical providers and medical staff
- Ensuring adequate testing before going live with patients
- Verifying expectations of warranty, support, and bug fix turn-around time from the technology vendor
- Providing internal training and communication regarding office workflow changes

In addition, technology has made tremendous progress in the past 10 years since the original mass move to electronic records began. Today's products have significantly more capabilities and better user interfaces. Companies are able to add new features and fix issues much faster, in many cases within 24 hours.

Typical Telemedicine Integration Approaches

When integrating telemedicine into a private practice or health system, the typical approaches are:

- Do it yourself (DIY) -- put together a mix of home-grown software with off-the-shelf hardware and software
- Hire a consultant or telemedicine integrator. Based on the requirements, the integrator will put together a custom telemedicine implementation using their own and off-the-shelf components
- Use a Telemedicine 2.0 software package

DIY is equivalent to hiring a consultant from a technical perspective. DIY uses an internal resource to do the work while hiring a consultant uses an external resource. The contractor may specialize in telemedicine integration, so they may be a better choice than DIY in some cases.

Both of the first two approaches, DIY and consultant, are the classic approaches to telemedicine implementation projects of the Telemedicine 1.0 era. They build the telemedicine solution from the ground up by using a mix of new and off-the-shelf components, and they tend to be narrowly customized for the requirements of the organization paying for the project. These approaches frequently use high-end dedicated videoconferencing software from vendors such as Cisco and Polycom. Take the example of a telemedicine consultation between a paramedic out in the field and the parent hospital's emergency department. Using a custom integration approach, the final solution will be tightly integrated with hospital's existing systems and equipment. The equipment that paramedics may use with the system will likely be limited, and the system will require future upgrades to integrate with newer equipment. These types of traditional implementation projects also tend to be tremendously expensive. They can only be undertaken by health systems and large practices with sufficient resources.

Most small and medium-sized practices implementing telemedicine are looking for a cost-effective solution that meets their needs and delivers a quality and efficient patient care experience. The best choice for these situations is to use a telemedicine software package from a telemedicine vendor. Most such off-the-shelf packages can be used with existing computers and mobile devices that physicians and patients already have, and require minimal setup or additional hardware costs. Some of the vendors offer risk-free trials, giving an opportunity for clinics to thoroughly review and test the software.

Most Telemedicine 2.0 software packages use software-as-a-service (SAAS) pricing model. That means these vendors charge for the usage of software at regular intervals, such as monthly. For details of the common pricing approaching, see the discussion on costs of telemedicine in the Store-and-Forward Telemedicine chapter.

Although many off-the-shelf telemedicine offering can be used as is, they often lack integration into the practice's existing systems. This means the telemedicine workflow is less than ideal. Luckily, most telemedicine vendors realize the importance of smooth clinic workflows around telemedicine, and they offer full clinic integration at an additional fee. The integration may either be a software module that was used or tested before, or it can be a new module developed specifically for the current customer. The quality and level of integration will vary from vendor to vendor.

Use a Vendor with Solid Technical Knowledge

When picking the right telemedicine vendor, it is important to pick a company with a solid technical foundation to complement your clinic's process and medical expertise. Many organizations that sell software technology solutions to healthcare industry are not technology companies – they are marketing companies. These software vendors focus most of their energies on pumping up the company brand and the supposed benefits of their product. Many do not have a technologist on their leadership team. Sometimes they may not even have a product -- they use artist rendered preview images of their product instead of the real thing. These marketing companies outsource their product development or hire low-level engineers to quickly slap something together. Their solutions are often not well architected, have tons of bugs, and don't use software industry best practices. If that wasn't bad enough, these companies also take a long time to add requested features and roll out much-needed fixes.

As a litmus test, ask your telemedicine vendor to implement a change or fix an issue, and see how long it takes them, as well as check out the quality of their work. This can be done during the risk-free trial before you're fully committed to the product. If they fail to impress, ask yourself whether you really want to trust a company that's likely run by inexperienced people?

This point is somewhat embarrassing to admit. We pride ourselves on working with the best people, but in our past we have worked with healthcare software providers who looked great at first impression but ended up being technically incompetent. We sure hope we learned our lesson. Here are some red flags when you're working with one of these:

- Constant pushback and negative feedback
- Long delays for trivial bug fixes, including delays before they can even provide a date for the bug fix
- Frequent schedule slips
- Low quality output
- Frequent excuses. For example, a critical engineer away on vacation the same week that a major feature rollout is expected
- The customer is not allowed to speak to engineers responsible for actual implementation
- Unmet expectations

Additionally, watch out for companies with deep hierarchies and long management chains. The reason is because product feature requirements must be communicated through multiple levels of management and may get lost in translation before they get to the actual engineers. The telemedicine vendor should help their clients get to the next level, and not be a "ball and chain" for progress. To gain technical confidence in your vendor, check out the resume of the vendor's Chief Technology Officer (CTO) or Lead Architect responsible for the telemedicine product.

- Does he have experience making products that people want?
- Does he have a deep and varied technology background?
- Has he led technical teams in the past?
- Can he get things done quickly?

As we alluded to earlier, a surprising number of healthcare technology providers are technically incompetent. (We speculate on the exact reasons for this later in this chapter.) It is no wonder the healthcare industry as a whole is having such basic issues as transferring patient data between systems. Working with such technically incapable companies results in frustration, destroyed expectations, going over budget, failed technology initiatives, and, for many medical providers, a vow to be wary about change in the future. Technical incompetency is one possible explanation why technical progress has been so slow in the healthcare space. In our current pool with many charlatans, there is a strong tendency to stick with the imperfect status quo. Some providers took a risk and leaped for a better tomorrow, but were disappointed by their chosen technology partner.

Some Vendors "Offer the Moon"

Many telemedicine vendors advertise that their software does everything -- it's the complete solution and the best thing since sliced bread. Do not take their word, but dig into the details. For example, some vendors state that they work with EMRs, and ask for a hefty fee to enable their EMR integration. However, there are different levels of integration. A full EMR integration should look up patients; update patient medication, allergies, and medical histories; synchronize with scheduling; and update the relevant sections of the patient record. However, simply claiming "we do EMR integration" may only mean that the vendor handles one of the many possible data transfer points.

Here is a common example of a trivial EMR integration. After a telemedicine visit, the telemedicine software creates a PDF of the patient encounter and stores it. Then, at night, the software runs a custom scheduled job to transfer the PDFs created that day to the EMR. Yes, it is EMR integration, but it is not a very good integration. If a vendor charges a hefty fee for EMR integration, make sure they give you all the needed functionality, and not just one trivial piece.

Some vendors "offering the moon" to potential customers are actually trying to sell solutions and features before they have even been created. In some cases, they sell the product before the engineers to build it have even been hired. Unfortunately, this is a common and legal marketing practice – companies try to test the market for the demand of their product by selling vaporware. If the demand is sufficient, then they will invest the funds to actually build it. In some cases, companies will try to charge the customer and then actually use those funds to build the product or feature.

Another factor justifying this sell-before-build marketing approach is the often-lengthy onboarding process for telemedicine – telemedicine deployments arc slow and rarely take quicker than a couple months. Most of that delay is not technical but administrative. Clinics must agree with and sign off on the care models, patient-visible content, and conditions to be treated by telemedicine. Physicians must sign off with their malpractice insurance provider. In addition, buy-in and feedback must be gathered from medical staff and interested parties, software training must be set up, etc. The wait required for this administrative process gives a competent telemedicine vendor time to actually implement and release an important feature for the customer, even if that feature was only a "pipe dream" when the product was originally sold to the customer.

The Customer-Vendor Relationship

The relationship with the telemedicine solution vendor is often more important than the actual provided technology. Even if one technology provider already has a magic feature that the other vendors are still working on, that doesn't guarantee that this vendor will still be a good fit for you 3, 6, or 12 months down the line. After all, if the practice integrates a new telemedicine workflow, they are not likely to switch unless the implementation is a complete failure or the vendor promised more than they could deliver. In either case, going through yet another implementation process is time-consuming and should be avoided if at all possible. The bottom line is that the technology vendor you choose should understand your business, strive to help you grow, and be extremely responsive to your needs and the needs of your patients. Choose a vendor that will last with you for the long term and help your practice grow successfully

Some telemedicine technology vendors trying to sell their software are also healthcare providers. That means they have their own provider network with physicians under contract, and they are delivering healthcare directly to the patients. They are looking to grow their direct-to-consumer services, bypassing the existing private clinics and specialists, and sending procedures only to their own providers. As you may have guessed, there is a conflict of interest here – these vendors are in direct competition with other medical providers that have their own clinics. Sure, their sales people will try to downplay this conflict as much as possible. But don't be fooled -- you should avoid buying software services from a company that is also trying to take your patients.

Now, this point warrants some additional explanation. Why would a healthcare provider try to sell their software to other healthcare providers? The simple answer is that the software has already been built, so why not also offer it up for sale. Several telemedicine software vendors in the industry started out building a product with a vision to connect any patient with any physician. This means when a patient opens up the vendor's app, they can pick to complete a telemedicine visit with any physician, even one who is really far away. Although this sounds great for patients, few physicians have signed up for these networks because these vendor networks don't offer enough value to established physician practices – they confuse existing and new patients, and they don't offer the individual physicians an opportunity to differentiate themselves. Patients are also not keen to get medical treatment directly through a telemedicine vendor. Oftentimes, a physician the patients know as well as physicians their friends recommend are not on these networks. What we've seen is that due to the slow adoption of this direct-to-consumer model, along with physician and patient pushback, many of these telemedicine vendors are now repackaging their software and offering to white-label it for individual physician practices. They're trying to have it both ways – offering health services to their own patients as well as to patients of other physicians.

Recommended Questions to Ask

Oftentimes, when selecting a new product or technology vendor, it is helpful to have plan of attack. Instead of going in and simply chatting with a potential vendor, it helps having a list of questions to ask. Then, after the conversations with all potential vendors are done, the vendors can be objectively compared based on their responses to the same set of questions. This is the same process we use at **md Portal** when interviewing employee candidates for open positions. This process adds a level of rigor to the selection procedure so that decisions are not clouded by first impressions. After all, we wouldn't want to hire an engineer to build a complex product when their only positive attribute is salesmanship.

Below are a few ideas for questions to ask a potential technology vendor:

- What is your experience with similar telemedicine deployments?
- Do you have references from existing customers?
- How do you handle data security and patient privacy? When was your last security audit and what changes did you make as a result?
- Can you scale with our practice – will you be able to handle more patients, physicians, and locations as our practice grows?
- What additional telemedicine features are on the horizon? When will we see them?
- What is the warranty? What is the customer support policy? Can we reach you on weekends or in the middle of the night?
- How big is your technical team working on this product? Who is on the team?
- How fast are bugs fixed?

Many healthcare facilities have an IT person or contract firm to handle tasks such as hosting the organization's web site and setting up computers in the office. This IT personnel will need to work closely with the telemedicine vendor. The existing IT staff also needs to be in sync with the vision of converting the clinic to a hybrid practice. This also means that the IT staff should be ready and available to provide help to the telemedicine technology vendor. Some questions to ask your internal IT staff before starting the telemedicine implementation:

- Will IT staff be available during the telemedicine implementation (no lengthy vacation plans)?
- Will existing IT stuff be sufficient to get the new system running and make any relevant updates to the existing systems, if needed?
- Are there other ongoing technology projects (website update, improving system integration, etc.) that may distract IT from assisting with the telemedicine implementation?

Before the telemedicine system goes live for patients and physicians, software must be fully tested. The software vendor must make a demo or trial version of the software system available to the clinic staff. Most telemedicine vendors provide a demo version of their solution or, even better, a risk-free trial, so that the clinic staff can use the system for testing purposes without a full commitment. It is important that as much functionality as possible be tested during the demo period, including focusing on any features that the clinic may not use right away, but plans to use in the near term or in the future. Most telemedicine systems support multiple user types, such as physicians, medical staff, organization admins, etc. During the demo period, the clinic staff should try using the software as each one of the relevant user types, in order to make sure the workflow and responsibilities fit into their current practice.

Attracting Top Software Talent to Healthcare

The inability to attract top software talent is a well known issue in the healthcare IT space. The healthcare industry is a highly regulated field with strict security requirements and many legal and procedural overheads. These overheads slow down the pace of innovation and make it more cumbersome for entrepreneurs to release new products or features. This also means software engineers cannot use some of the latest and greatest industry tools if those tools do not meet the strict healthcare regulation requirements. From our experience, most top software engineers prefer to move quickly and get things done, which is much easier to do in a non-regulated or non-medical space.

Another factor preventing many top software developers from switching to healthcare is their lack of in-depth knowledge regarding the process of medical patient treatment. For many, their only experience comes from their perspective as a patient, and they may not immediately comprehend the bigger picture of the medical treatment workflow. Ultimately, the top experts in healthcare are the medical providers who received many years of training. They are also the customers paying for many of the new and innovative software offerings. However, these busy medical professionals generally don't have time to regularly sit down with engineers and work through software development plans. Without a close working relationship between software developers and practicing physicians, any software product or new workflow "created in a vacuum" has a high chance of failure.

Luckily, several factors are changing the trend, including the overwhelming need for higher quality healthcare, the increasing importance of technology in healthcare, and the general perception that healthcare is broken and needs to be fixed. Engineers are increasingly beginning to view healthcare as an industry where their work may make the biggest impact. We hope that more and more engineers and talented software developers pick healthcare as the field to make their mark.

HIPAA, HITECH, and Health Information Security

In this chapter, we discuss patient privacy and the security safeguards that must be in place for telemedicine deployments. Although these security features are often implemented behind the scenes in telemedicine software products, they nevertheless require significant technical and administrative resources. We give a brief overview of the major government regulations and the common strategies to comply with them.

HIPAA is an acronym for the Health Insurance Portability and Accountability Act. It is pronounced similar to "hippo", and is often misspelled with two Ps instead of one. HIPAA was passed in 1996. The main goals of HIPAA are to:

- To protect health information
- To standardize electronic transactions
- Enforce the act by use of data breach notifications and financial penalties

HIPAA regulates the use and disclosure of PHI (Protected Health Information) by governing the "covered entities" and independent contractors that handle this data. The "covered entities" include healthcare clearinghouses, health plans, health insurers, and medical service providers. PHI is any information related to the individual's medical care, including medical record and payment history, which can be linked back to that individual. PHI comprises of two parts -- the medical care information and the identifying information. The unique data elements that can link back to the individual include: [37]

1. Name
2. Geographic locators such as address or latitude and longitude coordinates
3. Dates for significant personal events, such as birth, marriage, etc.
4. Phone numbers
5. Fax numbers
6. Email addresses
7. Social security numbers
8. Medical record numbers
9. Health plan beneficiary numbers, such as insurance member ID
10. Account numbers, such as bank account
11. Certificate/license numbers, such as driver's license
12. Vehicle identifiers and serial numbers, such as license plate number
13. Device identifiers and serial numbers, such as serial number of a computer
14. Website URLs, such as a link to a patient's social network profile
15. Internet Protocol (IP) address numbers, which can be used to identify the device

and location the person used to connect to the Internet
16. Biometric identifiers such as fingerprints, retinal images, etc.
17. Full face photo images or any images that can identify a person
18. Any other unique non-random number, characteristic, or code

Often, the term ePHI is also used, which stands for electronic PHI. For the purposes of modern telemedicine, where all data is stored and tracked digitally, all PHI is ePHI.

HITECH stands for Health Information Technology for Economic and Clinical Health Act. HITECH was passed in 2009 and intended to promote and broaden the adoption of health information technologies such as EHRs. HITECH expanded and improved HIPAA's privacy and security provisions by:

- Imposing new data breach notification requirements
- Extending HIPAA requirements to business associates of covered entities
- Adding specific provisions that should be covered in business associate agreements (BAAs)

What is HIPAA Compliance?

Every software vendor and telemedicine provider that is handling patient PHI must be HIPAA compliant. But what does that mean? HIPAA does not have a certifying body, so no government official will come in and put a HIPAA certification stamp on the product. Instead, the compliance is self-attested, which means any vendor can state that they are HIPAA compliant without really knowing if they are 100% HIPAA compliant. The fact that compliance is "in the eye of the beholder" and, at least partially, based on the organization's opinion, implies that different software vendors may put different amounts of effort towards their HIPAA security.

In contrast, other industries have specific certifications that must be received before an organization is allowed to do business in the sector. For example, the financial industry has PCI DSS (Payment Card Industry Data Security Standard) before handling credit card data. PCI certifications are received after the organization has completed the Common Security Framework (CSF) and a qualified security assessor approves the results.

If HIPAA compliance is self-attested, how does a telemedicine vendor prove that they are HIPAA compliant? There are three main approaches:

174

1. Self-assessments
2. Third Party Audit
3. Inheriting Proof

The three approaches are not exclusive, and may be combined with each other. Self-assessment is the easiest and least expensive path. Self-assessment means the telemedicine vendor completes their own internal assessment, and the proof is the supporting documentation coming out of this assessment, which should, at the minimum, include:

- Specific technology settings employed for all HIPAA requirements
- Specific policies in place for all HIPAA requirements

When the vendor achieves HIPAA compliance through self-assessment, the burden of trust falls on the buyer, the private practice or health system that is looking at the telemedicine solution. The buyer must trust the vendor, explicitly test the vendor by asking specific questions about HIPAA compliance, or perform a detailed review of the vendor's self-assessment documents. For the telemedicine vendor, this means the sales process is likely to consume more time, as well as increase the likelihood that the sale won't close.

Performing a third party HIPAA audit ahead of time is a quicker way for the telemedicine vendor to convince the buyer that the product is HIPAA compliant. However, third party audits are a lot more expensive, generally starting at $20,000. Typically, healthcare technology vendors don't do a third party audit until they have several major customers and are in the process of trying to scale their sales efforts. Of course, HIPAA auditors themselves are not regulated and their auditing procedures may vary widely. Still, having a third party stamp of approval and an audit report is the most reliable way for a vendor to prove their compliance.

The third approach is inhering proof. Most modern web software companies do not own their physical web servers, and instead host their applications on the servers of infrastructure providers such as Amazon Web Services (AWS). For telemedicine vendors, this means that the infrastructure providers must also handle PHI data, must have a business associate agreement (BAA), and must be HIPAA compliant. In effect, the HIPAA compliance responsibilities are shared between the telemedicine vendor and their infrastructure provider.

Some infrastructure providers take on a lot more HIPAA responsibilities and offer a lot more HIPAA compliance proof than others. For example, some infrastructure providers guarantee and provide encryption, system logging, vulnerability scanning, disaster recovery, and additional security services for healthcare applications. In addition, they provide proof of their own third party HIPAA audits that the telemedicine vendor and telemedicine vendor's customers can review.

Hence, inheriting proof can be a viable method for proving HIPAA compliance. It provides high quality proof for the areas handled by the infrastructure vendor. The infrastructure vendor's proof must be combined with telemedicine vendor's own proof for application concerns, such as application-level logging. However, the telemedicine vendor's own proof, either a self-assessment or a third party audit, as well as their HIPAA liabilities, would be much smaller in scope compared to a complete self-assessment.

Business Associate Agreements (BAAs) and Subcontractors

Business associates are companies that provide services to HIPAA's covered entities. As a reminder, covered entities include as healthcare clearinghouses, health plans, health insurers, and medical service providers. Telemedicine vendors are considered business associates because they handle protected health information (PHI). Handling PHI means processing, transmitting, storing, or interacting with the PHI data in some other way.

HIPAA requires business associates to have written contracts with covered entities that guarantee the safeguarding of PHI. In addition, business associates may have their own subcontractors that must also handle PHI, in which case HIPAA also requires the business associate and subcontractor to have a BAA. To take an example from the previous section, a telemedicine vendor may use an infrastructure provider such as AWS to store PHI. The telemedicine vendor must have a BAA with the infrastructure provider.

The specific requirement that subcontractors are also treated as business associates was added in the HITECH HIPAA Omnibus Rule of 2013. This recent requirement, in effect, creates chains of BAAs starting with covered entities and spreading to all the service providers that touch PHI. All of the companies in the chain must be HIPAA compliant. Below is the actual text from HIPAA's Code of Federal Regulations (45 CFR 164.308):

> (b)
> (1) **Business associate contracts and other arrangements.** A covered entity may permit a business associate to create, receive, maintain, or transmit electronic protected health information on the covered entity's behalf only if

the covered entity obtains satisfactory assurances, in accordance with § 164.314(a), that the business associate will appropriately safeguard the information. A covered entity is not required to obtain such satisfactory assurances from a business associate that is a subcontractor.

(2) A business associate may permit a business associate that is a subcontractor to create, receive, maintain, or transmit electronic protected health information on its behalf only if the business associate obtains satisfactory assurances, in accordance with§ 164.314(a), that the subcontractor will appropriately safeguard the information.

(3) **Implementation specifications: Written contract or other arrangement (Required).** Document the satisfactory assurances required by paragraph (b)(1) or (b)(2) of this section through a written contract or other arrangement with the business associate that meets

```
the applicable requirements of §
164.314(a).
```

BAAs, in addition to stating HIPAA guarantees, often also include details regarding the types of responsibilities the business associate takes on. Furthermore, these documents include details for data breach notifications and any penalties. Most companies have a standard BAA that they use with their vendors or customers. However, the BAAs must also be consistent with any other BAAs in the chain. For example, a telemedicine vendor selling to a private dermatology practice can't have a breach notification policy of 2 days if the BAA with their infrastructure provider has a breach notification policy of 5 days.

When using someone else's BAA, we strongly encourage you to read through the document in order to understand the legal responsibilities, and to ensure there are no conflicts. All telemedicine vendors must be willing to sign a BAA.

HIPAA Privacy Rule

The HIPAA Privacy and Security Rules go hand in hand with each other. The Privacy Rule provides definitions for covered entities, business associates, and PHI. In addition, it gives guidelines for health information disclosures and penalties for violators. In contrast, the Security Rule, to be discussed in the next section, provides specific technical requirements and policies for compliance.

Covered entities, as explained earlier, are the traditional businesses in healthcare, including healthcare clearinghouses, health plans, health insurers, and medical service providers, such as private clinics and hospitals. Business associates are the service providers, either individuals or organizations, which handle PHI. Telemedicine vendors are business associates.

PHI must be de-identified before being released to the public or released to another organization not part of the BAA chain. De-identification can be done through the Safe Harbor method, which removes all identifying information from the record, or through Expert Determination method, using a statistician to ensure that any single individual in the data is unlikely to be identified.

There are also cases when PHI can be disclosed as is, without de-identification. Below are the most common allowed reasons for PHI disclosure:

- Upon individual request – with written permission from the individual requesting disclosure of their own health information

- For medical treatment – exchanging information between providers who are treating the person's medical condition(s)
- For collecting payment, whether from health insurers or other payers
- For operations, including administrative functions and medical education
- For legal reasons, such as a request for information from a judicial court

Whenever handling PHI, the tenant of "minimum necessary use" must be followed. This means that individuals and organizations should not disclose more PHI that absolutely necessary. For example, when checking patient's eligibility for a telemedicine follow-up with their insurance, it should not be necessary to disclose details from an unrelated procedure done 10 years ago.

Patients must be notified of their rights. This is commonly done through privacy policies that patients must acknowledge whenever receiving medical treatment.

The Office of Civil Rights (OCR), which is part of the U.S. Department of Health & Human Services (HHS), enforces HIPAA rules. Penalties for disclosing or illegally obtaining PHI include fines as well as imprisonment.

HIPAA Security Rule

The Security Rule spells out the specific technical requirements and policies necessary for HIPAA compliance. That said, some of the wordings in the Security Rule are open to interpretation. The Security Rule covers the following safeguard areas needed for compliance:

- Administrative
- Physical
- Technical

The administrative area covers the policies that must be in place for an organization to comply with HIPAA. The descriptions of the required policies make up most of the content of the Security Rule. One of the most important HIPAA policies for an organization is the regular **Risk Assessment**.

The risk assessment is a regular procedure done by the organization which:

- Documents the overall architecture of the PHI data flow
- Identifies areas of risk for PHI data breaches
- Puts in place mitigation plans for the identified risks

Risk assessment is often the first procedure done by the organization on its path to HIPAA compliance. Documenting the overall architecture means taking an inventory of all the systems belonging to the organization, and mapping out how and whether those systems handle PHI. The areas of risk may include anything from a stolen laptop to a malicious hacker breaking into the organization's systems. For each area of risk, the likelihood and impact should be assessed. For each risk item, a mitigation strategy should be in place. Not everything will be 100% mitigated. Some risks may not be mitigated completely, depending on their likelihood, the difficulty of implementing the fix, and available organization resources.

Other administrative policies that must be in place to achieve HIPAA compliance include:

- Workforce authorization, supervision, and termination policies, including a sanction policy for non-compliant workforce members
- Security awareness and training policies
- Security incident (breach) policies
- Contingency planning policies, including data backup and disaster recovery plans

The physical safeguards covered in HIPAA's Security Rule apply to physically accessible devices for a covered entity or business associate. The policies and implementations associated with the physical safeguards must be documented. They physical safeguard areas are:

- Facility access controls
- Employee workstations
- Device and media controls (mini USB drives, CDs, etc.)

The facility access controls should limit or eliminate unauthorized physical access to the company's electronic information systems. Some members of the organization may not need physical access to the systems, and, hence, should not be allowed access. Physical access to the facility may be controlled by methods such as:

- Door locks
- Electronic access control systems
- Security officers
- Video monitoring

For employee workstations, only employees that require PHI access must be allowed access to workstations containing PHI. Methods to safeguard workstation access include:

- Password protection
- Automatic logoff after a period of time
- Privacy screens, which are panels that limit the computer screen's angle of

vision so that onlookers cannot easily see what the employee is working on
- Encrypted hard drives

Device and media controls apply to portable media that can be removed from the premises or moved around at the facility, such as computer hard drives, CDs, DVDs, digital memory sticks, and others. When reusing or disposing such devices, any PHI on them must be completely removed. The location of devices containing PHI must be tracked.

One last point to make about the security rule is that not all implementation specifications listed in the security rule are required. Some are marked **addressable**. An addressable specification means the organization may do one of the following:

- Implement the specification as written
- Implement an alternative specification that addresses the same issue
- Do not implement the specification because it is not reasonable or necessary

The implementation may not be reasonable because the cost of implementation may be more than company can afford. The implementation may not be necessary depending on the type of company. For example, an employee termination procedure is not necessary if the organization is a one-person sole proprietorship. If the specification was not implemented, the covered entity or business associate must document this decision and the reasons behind it.

Data Breaches

A data breach is an unauthorized exposure of PHI. A breach can occur by accident, like the example of an employee forgetting a media device with PHI in a restaurant. Or, a breach can occur because a 3rd party forcibly removed information, such as a hacker or identify thief. According to an info graphic published by RockHealth [38], common reasons for breaches include the following, with the most common listed first:

- Lost or stolen computing device
- Employee mistake or unintentional accident
- 3rd party mistake
- Criminal attack
- Technical system glitch
- Malicious insider
- Intentional non-malicious employee action

After a data breach, the business associate must notify their customer of the breach. Their customer is either a covered entity or another business associate. The notice shall include the list of individuals whose PHI was affected. The exact process and timing requirements for the notification are typically spelled out in the business associate agreement (BAA) between the two companies. HIPAA allows a maximum of 60 days for notifications, with the caveat that any delay must be explainable with sufficient evidence. Either the business associate or the covered entity must notify the specific individual patients whose data was disclosed.

Future of Telemedicine: Telemedicine 3.0 and Beyond

As the Chief Technology Officer at md Portal, I look at the technology trends, figure out where they are heading, and estimate their impact on the future of the company. The 1924 radio doctor article from "Radio News" [9] is a great example of visualizing the future. The article depicts a patient visit using television, along with real-time heartbeat and temperature sensors. Today, this type of patient visit is done regularly, combining real-time video telemedicine with remote patient monitoring. Thus, just like that article, in this chapter we will speculate on the future advancements in telemedicine, healthcare, and related technologies. At md Portal, we're working around the clock to bring many of these ideas to reality.

As we mentioned in the introduction, the "2.0" moniker is associated with Web 2.0 and related technologies. At the time of this writing, there is no consensus on what Web 3.0 will be, beyond the basic understanding that it will be an evolution beyond Web 2.0. Similarly, when discussing Telemedicine 3.0, we will speak of the general evolution of telemedicine beyond the current technologies and implementations. It is also worth noting that Telemedicine 2.0 is still in the "early majority" stage of the innovation curve, and it will take a few more years for it to be adopted by most of the healthcare industry. Many people still consider telemedicine a new technology. Thus, some of the ideas we cover in this chapter may be implemented as soon as the next several years, and be rolled out as upgrades to the current suite of Telemedicine 2.0 products.

Remote Monitoring for Everyone

Remote monitoring, as covered in the Remote Monitoring chapter, is currently used for postoperative recovery, special conditions such as diabetes and heart disease, and for the elderly. As innovations in wearable sensors and related technologies continue, we expect everyone, even the healthy, to be able to use basic remote monitoring technologies.

In the future, people may choose to be remotely monitored their entire life, starting at birth. Imagine the 9-1-1 operators immediately seeing all your vital signs on their screen during an emergency. In addition, physician can use remote monitoring history to optimize the patient's treatment plan. When visiting a physician with a medical issue, your medical provider may select a therapy that has a high success rate for patients with your remote monitoring profile.

Wearable sensors are already becoming cheaper, more user friendly, and inconspicuous. For example, the Apple Watch, released in April of 2015, is able to monitor activity and heart rate. The watch synchronizes this monitoring data into the Apple HealthKit infrastructure, from where it can be retrieved by other applications, such as third party telemedicine apps. As the wearable trend continues, simple devices such as watches, armbands, and body-contact stick-on pads will gain more functionality and integrate additional sensors, including blood oxygen and glucose monitoring. Smart clothing, containing sensors, will also become prevalent.

Today, many physicians don't see sufficient value in popular activity monitoring devices such as Fitbit. Although the fact that the patient is using a Fitbit tracker suggests that the patient is motivated to maintain or improve their health, the actual data provided by these devices, in the opinion of many medical providers, does not offer sufficient medical significance today.

One key that is missing in today's remote monitoring devices is analytics, specifically search and intelligent alert capabilities. Patients and physicians must be able to perform intelligent searches on the data. The searches must take into account multiple variables. In the future, the telemedicine systems will be able to immediately answer many common questions. A couple example questions are:

- What are my typical vitals when temperature is 90°F and I've been outside for longer than 10 minutes?
- What is my peak blood pressure when I fly on a plane?

Ready availability of data from such queries will allow health systems run statistical analysis on patient populations and correlate remote monitoring with diagnoses and treatment plans. In addition to intelligent search, future remote monitoring systems will have intelligent alerts which can be directed to the patient's physician, directly to 9-1-1, or to someone else. For example, if the system senses abnormal vital signs, a likely heart attack, stroke, seizure, or serious wound, 9-1-1 can be automatically contacted. The patient's vitals and location will be automatically sent to the dispatcher. If the patient was driving at the time of the event, their car will be alerted to pull off to the side of the road.

People's surroundings will also have sensors, and data from these external sensors can be piped into the patient's main remote monitoring system. For example, in the near future, we'll have cars with temperature, heart rate, and respiration sensors. Smart homes will also have these sensors along with many others. Future home floors, mirrors, chairs, beds, and showers will take body temperature, weight, and other important body measurements. Smart homes will also be able to monitor the health condition of any guest in addition to the main occupants. When urinating in the toilet, an automatic urine test will be done to check how the person's kidneys are functioning and if they are at a risk for diabetes.

Now, all this talk of "health monitoring everywhere" may bring up images of Big Brother. Will the government, insurance companies, or other corporations use this data for nefarious means, such as exerting control over the human population? These are valid concerns. In many ways, they are similar to the contemporary concerns raised about privacy of today's electronic medical records. We saw the EMR concerns increase as the healthcare industry was transitioning to EMR systems. We expect that all remote monitoring data of the future to be classified as protected information, with appropriate safeguards in place. Additional laws and procedures may need to be put in place. For example, people may need to opt-in before external sensors, such as those in public buildings, are allowed to save their health data.

Full Medical Exam from Home

In the future, patients will be able to do their early wellness visit from the comfort of their own home, or from a convenient location such as a grocery store or school. A typical physical exam includes:

- Head and neck exam
- Abdominal exam
- Neurological exam
- Cardiovascular exam
- Pulmonary exam
- Psychiatric exam
- Dermatological exam
- Exam of the extremities
- Male or female-specific exams
- Laboratory tests

The first technical component needed for the exam is the full view of the patient. Telemedicine exam rooms, such as those in schools or rural clinics, will already have the proper video equipment. At home, the patients will either use a dedicated video setup or re-purpose their existing cameras for telemedicine. Many homes already have high definition security cameras. As the camera quality improves, these security cameras could double for telemedicine visits. In addition, the telemedicine systems will support multiple simultaneous camera feeds – cameras will be located at different angles around the patient to give the medical provider a full body view.

Taking it a step further, telemedicine software will be able to take the video feeds from multiple angles and reconstruct a 3-D version of the patient. This way the examining physician, instead of looking at several separate video streams, could view the patient in 3-D, including zooming into the patient's body parts as needed. Several sections of the exam will be automated, such as full-body mole checks, and medical provider will only focus on the anomalies and outliers flagged by the software.

Special equipment and cameras will be used for head, neck and other exams. The equipment will either be cheap enough where the patient will simply order the telemedicine kit online, or the patient will rent the sterilized equipment for use during the exam, much like DVDs can be rented via mail today. The equipment will be user friendly enough where the patients can use it themselves without professional help. Alternatively, a second person, such as the patient's spouse or parent, could handle the equipment.

Some of exam portions are too complex for today's technologies, such as abdominal, pelvic, and prostate exams. In the future, special equipment will be developed for these exams, such as haptic technologies, which we will address in the next section. Alternatively, proxy tests will be used that provide equivalent clinical information. For example, today, prostate-specific antigen blood tests are often used instead of the traditional manual prostate exam.

The full telemedicine medical exam requires vitals and laboratory tests. Patient vitals will be taken with standard remote monitoring devices. Blood and urine will be collected into miniature containers and sent off to the clinical lab by mail or drone.

The patient will be able to use real-time or store-and-forward telemedicine for this wellness visit. For real-time, the patient will have a live video feed with the medical provider, nurse, or a medical assistant to guide them through the process. With store-and-forward, patient will do all the steps themselves, using an interactive questionnaire and instructions, and the medical provider will review the results at their convenience.

Haptic Technologies and Future of Telesurgery

Haptic technologies provide physical feedback to the user by trying to recreate the sense of touch, motion, vibration, and other tactile senses. Haptic technologies are being used in today's telesurgery systems. This book has not focused on telesurgery because today's telesurgery is only being used for specific procedures, and we do not consider it a Telemedicine 2.0 technology. However, the impact and scope of telesurgery and other haptic technologies will considerably expand in the upcoming Telemedicine 3.0 era.

In the future, telesurgery at long distances will be extremely common. For example, the surgery patient may be in Hawaii while physician operating the surgery robot may be in Cleveland, Ohio. Of course, local surgical staff will also be on site with the patient in case of emergencies. Such an arrangement will allow surgeons (or teams of surgeons) to specialize in very specific types of surgeries. This means that most patients will be able to receive surgeries from the top experts in the field without enduring unnecessary travel or time delays.

In addition, the surgery robots will be sufficiently cheap and mobile so that they could be transported to the patient's location. For example, the robot could be taken to a nursing home, a prison, or even to a patient's home. Then, along with on-site staff present in case of emergencies, the remote surgeon will perform the surgery at the patient's location.

Besides telesurgery, simpler haptic devices will be available for regular physical examinations. The idea behind medical haptic devices is that the physician will be able to physically feel a patient's body area from a distance, whether abdomen, skin area, or some other part. One way it may work is the following.

Patient will put the device on the area of the examination. The device will contain many sensors, including tactile, pressure, temperature, visual, sound, and others. The information from these sensors will either be recorded or streamed to the remote operator. The haptic device will also have the ability to apply pressure, achieving the examination feedback loop – the operator will apply pressure to a specific area and watch for the response from the sensors. It is worth noting that the patient themselves could do their own physical examination using such a device by following instructions, and the medical provider can review the results later. In the extreme case, this exam could even be done completely by a computer.

Today, touch screens for mobile devices such as the iPhone and tablets drive much of the progress in tactile sensors and haptic technologies. Soon, mobile touch screens will distinguish multiple levels of pressure as well as provide feedback. Telemedicine devices will then quickly adopt these technologies. Imagine squeezing the patient's skin from your mobile tablet, seeing the results, and feeling the tension.

Artificial Intelligence

Artificial intelligence (AI) is the ability of computers to perform tasks that typically require human intelligence. The IBM Watson machine is the poster child for using artificial intelligence in the healthcare space. After gaining fame on the television quiz show *Jeopardy!*, Watson went into the healthcare space to assist with clinical decisions in places such as the University of Texas MD Anderson Cancer Center. [39]

Going forward, IBM Watson and similar systems will become more and more powerful. These technologies will be used by telemedicine systems to suggest patient diagnosis and treatments. By examining the patient questionnaires, images, videos, past patient history, and medical literature, the AI systems will be able to make differential diagnosis and treatment recommendations to medical providers. The AI systems will be able to interact with patients by asking them additional questions and recommending further tests to narrow down the diagnosis.

Now, you may wonder, if the AI systems will become so powerful, will we even need doctors? The short answer is yes. There will always be tasks that cannot be done by computers. Since the advent of computers, many tasks have been delegated to or improved by machines, such as factory assembly work, simulations of complex biological systems, and airplane landings. These improvements freed up many humans to focus on more complex and higher value work. In a similar way, AI systems of the future may be able to correctly diagnose and treat 90% or more of medical conditions, but there we always be corner cases and new, never before seen circumstances that will require human input. In addition, as humans live longer and longer, the elderly will require new and innovative approaches to treatment than the rest of the population, which AI may not be able to handle.

In the future, AI will be combined with remote monitoring – the patient, in effect, will have a continuous real-time medical exam performed on them as they go about in their daily life. The AI system may, occasionally, ask the patient a one-off question about their intentions, mood, or something else to help calibrate itself. This system will be powerful for preventative health, since it will be able to offer real-time suggestions and warnings. If a medical problem is suspected, the system may automatically send off the patient's vitals and diagnosis recommendation to the patient's medical provider.

Strong AI, defined as AI that is as intelligent as a person, is widely considered to be the last invention that humans will need to make. The reason is because once AI is as smart as a person, it can create another AI that is even smarter than itself, and so on and so forth. Many experts doubt if such an invention will happen in the foreseeable future. One thing is for sure, by the time strong AI arrives, medicine and telemedicine will be completely different from what we know today.

Conclusion

In this book, we covered the past, the present, and the future of telemedicine. Many medical practices have already transitioned to telemedicine and many others are actively considering it. Within several years, we expect most medical practices to use some form of telemedicine 2.0 as part of their services. There are challenges to telemedicine implementations, and we tried our best not to downplay or gloss over any of them. Telemedicine 2.0 offers huge advantages, patient demand, and the need to get it done and get it done right. At **md Portal**, we're striving to push the ball forward and make visits for all routine medical conditions available via telemedicine.

For questions, comments, or suggestions for future editions of this book, feel free to contact the author at victor@mdportal.com

References

[1] Susan D. Hall. (2015, May) Rapid growth projected for global telemedicine market. [Online]. http://www.fiercehealthit.com/story/rapid-growth-projected-global-telemedicine-market/2015-05-20

[2] American Telemedicine Association. (2015, Aug.) What is Telemedicine? [Online]. http://www.americantelemed.org/about-telemedicine/what-is-telemedicine

[3] Gunther Eysenbach, "Medicine 2.0: Social Networking, Collaboration, Participation, Apomediation, and Openness," *J Med Internet Res*, vol. 10, no. 3, p. e22, Aug. 2008, http://www.jmir.org/2008/3/e22/.

[4] Justin Caba. (2014, Jan.) Doctor's Appointment Average Wait Time 18.5 Days Across 15 Cities: Boston Patients Wait Average 72 Days For Dermatologist. [Online]. http://www.medicaldaily.com/doctors-appointment-average-wait-time-185-days-across-15-cities-boston-patients-wait-average-72-days

[5] Rashid Bashshur, PhD and Gary W. Shannon, *History of Telemedicine: Evolution, Context, and Transformation*. New Rochelle, NY: Mary Ann Liebert, 2009.

[6] Marilyn J. Field, *Telemedicine: A Guide to Assessing Telecommunications in Health Care*. Washington, D.C.: National Academy, 1996.

[7] John Plunkett. (2012, July) Decline of the phone call: Ofcom shows growing trend for text communication. [Online]. http://www.theguardian.com/technology/2012/jul/18/ofcom-report-phone-calls-decline

[8] Erin McCann. (2012, Aug) Getting the fax straight. [Online]. http://www.healthcareitnews.com/news/getting-fax-straight?single-page=true

[9] FIPS, "The Radio Doctor--Maybe," *Radio News*, p. 1406+, Apr 1924, http://www.americanradiohistory.com/Archive-Radio-News/20s/Radio-News-1924-04-R.pdf.

[10] Teresa Wang. (2014, June) The Future of Biosensing Wearables. [Online]. http://rockhealth.com/2014/06/future-biosensing-wearables/

[11] Lauren Gensler. (2015, May) Fitbit Files For IPO, Reveals Surprising Profits. [Online]. http://www.forbes.com/sites/laurengensler/2015/05/07/fitbit-files-for-ipo/

[12] American Medical Association. (2003, June) Opinion 5.026 - The Use of Electronic Mail. [Online]. http://www.ama-assn.org/ama/pub/physician-resources/medical-ethics/code-medical-

ethics/opinion5026.page?

[13] Jacqueline Bain. (2015, Apr.) Physician Communications: Considerations for Using Text Messages and Social Media. [Online]. http://www.avvo.com/legal-guides/ugc/physician-communications-considerations-for-using-text-messages-and-social-media

[14] (2015, Aug.) Terra medica Teleradiology center. [Online]. http://www.tcleradiology-center.eu/en/technology-2

[15] John D. Whited, "Summary of the Status of Teledermatology Research," Teledermatology Special Interest Group American Telemedicine Association, Durham, 2015.

[16] Anne Montgomery. (2015, Mar.) Telemedicine Provides Better Care and More Patient Engagement; Challenges Remain. [Online]. http://altarum.org/about/news-and-events/telemedicine-provides-better-care-and-more-patient-engagement-challenges-remain

[17] Katie Wike. (2014, May) Patients Satisfied With Telehealth For Follow-up Care. [Online]. http://www.healthitoutcomes.com/doc/patients-satisfied-with-telehealth-for-follow-up-care-0001

[18] MD Barron H. Lerner. (2014, Nov.) When Patients Don't Follow Up. [Online]. http://well.blogs.nytimes.com/2014/11/1

3/when-patients-dont-follow-up/?_r=1

[19] Health IT Dashboard. (2015, Apr.) Office-based Health Care Professional Participation in the CMS EHR Incentive Programs. [Online]. http://dashboard.healthit.gov/quickstats/pages/FIG-Health-Care-Professionals-EHR-Incentive-Programs.php

[20] Dike Drummond. (2013, Nov.) 9 Reasons Physicians Hate EMR - The 2013 RAND Study. [Online]. http://www.thehappymd.com/blog/bid/351428/9-Reasons-Physicians-Hate-EMR-The-2013-RAND-Study

[21] Mark Friedberg, Francis J. Crosson, and Michael Tutty. (2014, Mar.) Physicians' Concerns About Electronic Health Records: Implications And Steps Towards Solutions. [Online]. http://healthaffairs.org/blog/2014/03/11/physicians-concerns-about-electronic-health-records-implications-and-steps-towards-solutions/

[22] American Telemedicine Association. (2015, May) Milestone – Most States Now Have Telehealth Parity Laws. [Online]. http://www.americantelemed.org/news-landing/2015/05/27/milestone-most-states-now-have-telehealth-parity-laws

[23] Home Depot. (2015, Sep.) TELADOC – TALK TO A DOCTOR 24/7/365. [Online]. https://secure.livethehealthyorangelife.co

m/health_care/teladoc

[24] Teladoc. (2015, Apr.) Teladoc moves to block Medical Board rule that would restrict health care access for millions of Texans. [Online]. http://www.teladoc.com/news/2015/04/29/teladoc-moves-to-block-medical-board-rule-that-would-restrict-health-care-access-for-millions-of-texans/

[25] David Heitz. (2014, Nov.) Telepsychiatry Is Taking Over in Places Shrinks Can't Reach. [Online]. http://www.healthline.com/health-news/telepsychiatry-in-places-shrinks-can-t-reach-112914

[26] Lisa B Marshall. (2015, Aug.) How Fast Do I Speak? (Update). [Online]. http://www.lisabmarshall.com/2014/01/23/how-fast-do-i-speak-update/

[27] Elizabeth Bernstein. (2012, Oct.) Why We Are So Rude Online. [Online]. http://www.wsj.com/articles/SB10000872396390444459240457803035178440514 8

[28] Donald K. Cherry and Susan M. Schappert. (2014, Nov.) QuickStats: Percentage of Mental Health–Related* Primary Care† Office Visits, by Age Group — National Ambulatory Medical Care Survey, United States, 2010. [Online]. http://www.cdc.gov/mmwr/preview/mmwrhtml/mm6347a6.htm

[29] Amy Lerman. (2014, Nov.) CMS Expands

Telehealth Reimbursement in New Rule. [Online]. http://www.techhealthperspectives.com/2014/11/05/cms-expands-telehealth-reimbursement-in-new-rule/

[30] Neil Chesanow. (2014, Jan.) Can We Get Patients to Be More Compliant? [Online]. http://www.medscape.com/viewarticle/819317

[31] (2015, Aug.) InfluxDB. [Online]. https://influxdb.com/

[32] Atul Gawande, *Being Mortal: Medicine and What Matters in the End*. New York: Metropolitan Books, Henry Hold and Company, LLC, 2014.

[33] Brian Dolan. (2013, Mar.) Does Fitbit's WiFi-enabled Aria scale need FDA clearance? [Online]. http://mobihealthnews.com/20765/does-fitbits-wifi-enabled-aria-scale-need-fda-clearance/

[34] U.S. Department of Health and Human Services, Food and Drug Administration, Center for Devices and Radiological Health, Office of Device Evaluation. (2015, July) Intent to Exempt Certain Unclassified, Class II, and Class I Reserved Medical Devices from Premarket Notification Requirements. Guidance for Industry and Food and Drug Administration Staff. [Online]. http://www.fda.gov/downloads/MedicalDevices/DeviceRegulationandGuidance/Guida

nceDocuments/UCM407292.pdf

[35] Detlev H. Smaltz and Eta S. Berner, *The Executive's Guide to Electronic Health Records.*: Health Administration Press, 2007.

[36] Catherine M. Desroches et al., "Electronic Health Records in Ambulatory Care — A National Survey of Physicians," *New England Journal of Medicine*, vol. 359, July 2008.

[37] (2015, Apr.) OSHPD - Committee for the Protection of Human Subjects. [Online]. http://www.oshpd.ca.gov/Boards/CPHS/HIPAAIdentifiers.pdf

[38] RockHealth. (2013, Mar) 94% of Healthcare Organizations Breached. [Online]. http://rockhealth.com/wp-content/uploads/2013/03/34f9a961f56ac6d3013d8b1bd266ef3b96fee194.png

[39] MD Anderson. (2013, Oct.) MD Anderson Taps IBM Watson to Power "Moon Shots" Mission. [Online]. http://www.mdanderson.org/newsroom/news-releases/2013/ibm-watson-to-power-moon-shots-.html

About the Author

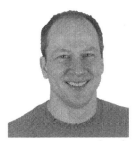

Victor Lyuboslavsky is the Chief Technology Officer at mdPortal.com, one of the leading telemedicine providers. He has worked with numerous private practices from dermatology to primary care to help them transition to telemedicine, optimize their workflows, and deliver a better and more efficient patient experience. Victor is a member of the American Telemedicine Association (ATA) and Healthcare Information and Management Systems Society (HIMSS). He is recognized as one of the leading authorities on telemedicine technologies.

Victor has founded multiple successful companies, including several in health care, and has over 15 years of total experience in high tech leadership roles. He holds an MS in Electrical and Computer Engineering from the University of Texas at Austin and an MBA from UMass Amherst.

Twitter: @lyuboslavsky

Made in the USA
Lexington, KY
22 May 2018